As Light as a Feather

OR

An Uncommon Affair

by

Dr. F. Walton Avery, MD, MTS

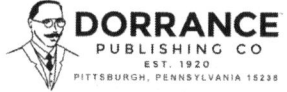
DORRANCE
PUBLISHING CO
EST. 1920
PITTSBURGH, PENNSYLVANIA 15235

Dorrance Publishing Co
585 Alpha Drive
Suite 103
Pittsburgh, PA 15238
Visit our website at *www.dorrancebookstore.com*

ISBN: 978-1-4809-2726-1
eISBN: 978-1-4809-2864-0

"Don't go around tonight,
Well, it's bound to take your life,
There's a bad moon on the rise."[1]

"...life turns on a dime..."[2]

"...what are human beings that you are mindful of them, mortals that you care for them?"[3]

"We eventually experience pleasure in doing good acts and pain in doing bad acts, thus develop the internal habitual disposition to be moral."[4]

"The real perspective here is that these are not 'Black Swan' events or one-off things that are fundamentally unpredictable. These are known patterns."[5]

---

[1] Credence Clearwater Revival: "Bad Moon Rising" (chorus).
[2] King, Stephen: 11/22/63 (New York, Scribner, 2011)
[3] Psalm 8:4 (NRSV)
[4] Chaumiere, Richard: What's It All About (Sonoma: Wisdom House Press, p.106)
[5] Nathan Wolfe: "Weekend Confidential: Alexandra Wolfe" (WSJ, December 13-14, 2014, p. C17)

PREFACE

The following is a fictional discourse between Stephen King[6], the writer, and yours truly, the reader; discussing whether or not we have control over our lives. Is maintaining control over our lives like that baseball that seems to settle on its own in the outfield grass?

R: "In '11/22/63' you used the expression, "life turns on a dime," on more than one occasion and often at the end of a paragraph. A casual reader might just pass that by with only a thought, 'the vicissitudes and happenings of life can occur on a rather thin turn of events.' Is that what you meant?"

W: "Not necessarily vicissitudes, which I presume you are using a negative sense, because there are positive changes that seem to occur on what you call a 'thin turn of events.' That's what I meant when I said, 'Sometimes toward us, but more often it spins away...' It is to say that life's events may seem (or interpreted as) positive and others may seem (or interpreted as) negative, and I think you can see that which way the dime turns depends, not totally, but at least partially, on one's own gestalt and/or belief system.

R: "Are these occurrences isolated events or what one might call the constant back and forth of life?"

---

[6] I sent a request/notification to Scribner Publishers concerning the Prologue which utilizes a fictional discourse between Stephen King, the writer, and me the reader. I received no response from the publisher.

W: "At the time of an event, it may seem isolated, as you call it; but, upon reflection, it is not isolated, but simply part of the ebb and flow of life, as in 'living life."

R: Life is living and living is life?"

W: "Ah, the great paradox of existentialism: why are we here or what does it mean to exist."

R: "Back to the expression, 'life turns on a dime,' is it just a poetic metaphor for the events of life that each of us experiences, or is it the answer to the question, 'Can I understand why things happen to me?' Or does it simply refer to the fact that things are going to happen to me which I have no control over?"

W: "All of the above. When it is all said and done, we have to ask, 'Can I differentiate between things happening as a result of fate (undetermined cause) and things happening as a result of our own volition?'

R: It is the question for the ages, but one cannot get around the fact that it all may be predetermined by the genes we have inherited from our parents or by the interaction between these genes and the factors of the environment."

I submitted a written request to the publisher, Scribner and Company, for permission to use this material from Stephen King, but I received no response.

W: "Yes, that is true, stating that each of us is greatly influenced by where and how we live, what we eat and breathe, and what persons or animals that we interact with. It is clear to me that the environment can alter our genetic makeup; so fate or not, we are the victims of our choices."

R: "So we have come full circle in the examination of life and how we live it. Life does turn on a dime, but life remains in our hands. Can we say that the circle is complete without a reference to God?"

W: "I think it is critical to understand that we have been given the blessing or the curse of freewill and it can clearly be either. You can see references to the God-gene; you can read arguments that cite the underlying morality of the creation. But still, whether for good or evil, the human being sometimes makes decisions that appear to be random and not reflecting God or morality."

R: "Therefore, the ball that settles in the outfield grass bespeaks both intentionality and randomness. We are like that ball: surely someone will come along and put us back into play. From the dull crack of the bat to the presence of the second baseman, the ball will inevitably find a home. No doubt the ballpark and the players represent the gestalt of life. The odds are for us, and God does more than throw the dice. At least we hope so. Yes, we have to keep on keeping on, yet we cannot ignore the silence of a feather when it falls to the ground.

A Note to the Reader

Before you read any further, please be aware that this novel is predominantly about the relationship that develops between a man and a woman—aspects of this relationship are emotional, mental, spiritual or physical. Eventually, any relationship between a man and a woman becomes complex and exhibits all of these aspects. In seemingly normal couples, by implication, this relationship will eventually involve sex. And, again by implication, there are frequent episodes in this book that occur as a result of sex between men and women. This book also examines the relationship between preadolescent and adolescent boys who gathered in small groups for what they call sexual games. Does this activity get out of bounds? Yes, maybe, depending on who is speaking, for separate twosomes may gather in a private location for autoerotic sex. It is evident, however, that none of this early "homosexual" activity carries over into the late adolescent period or adulthood.

At first, this story is about baseball and other aspects of life, but the subsequent and most profound part of this tale is the chief protagonist's personal remembrances related to an obsession with heterosexual sex. Like alcoholism and other forms of addiction—therapy or not—physical obsession with the opposite sex remains with the afflicted victim for life. No doubt, the intensity of such an obsession can be altered up or down by the will of the victim. Such an alteration,

DR. F. WALTON AVERY, MD, MTS

of course, requires energy and late in life the obsession may lose its steam. Thus, sex eventually becomes secondary for the chief protagonist, but it still casts a shadow over his life. He will go to his grave knowing there is, like the apostle Paul, a "catch" in his side. It is not stated or shown with clarity how "lust" can be differentiated from "love," but, on the other hand, it may be true that one cannot ever differentiate between the two because one is part and parcel of the other. As the events of the novel become narrowed down to an "Uncommon Affair" between our two main characters, we can witness the development of a relationship where lust is recognized for what it is, but love is the force and foundation of the affair and is more powerful than life itself.

x

CHAPTER ONE

"Wasp"

Jackie Moreland, our chief character and male protagonist—looking into the mirror and creating a selfie—has always been a white male and has always acted like one—never acted or dressed like a woman and never acted or dressed like any non-white person. He has always been a Protestant Christian but never a Catholic, Jew, or Muslim. He has always been from the American South, saddled—noted by some people not from the South—with a typical southern accent and mindset. Finally, he is an Anglo-Saxon, and, putting all these characteristics together, he is a "WASP."

The following discussion about the female wasp is as much about the human and animal reactions that are either offensive or defensive. The female wasp may sting a victim and, immediately, the injected venom elicits a stinging pain. Without the application of a neutralizing base material, the site of the sting becomes red and swollen and remains painful; there is also an immediate allergic reaction and the victim may want to scratch it, but woe unto her, if she scratches it and the stinger is still in the wound.

A sting from a threatened insect is a very uncomfortable reminder that all animals have a defense mechanism that protect them from harm. Unfortunately, and not so infrequently, the difference between

1

a defensive and offensive reaction may be blurred and a victim may be hurt or even killed. This is particularly true with respect to the higher animals and human beings. In comparison with, or contrast to, the wasp, what is the human being that we speak of? What is the human being's purpose in life? Is that purpose for good or evil or both? What is it that drives the human to perform an evil act? When or why does a defensive action become an offensive action? What is it that allows the human to know the difference between a good and an evil act? Is it an inchoate trait or a learned phenomenon or both?

Jackie is a man: as he has lived his life, he has finally realized he is a heterosexual man. He knows the difference between right and wrong and acts on that knowledge nine times out of ten or better. But even knowing the difference between right and wrong, he still may think wrong and do wrong. As with any human being, it is inherent in his makeup that he is capable of thinking about and/or performing an act that is wrong. Before we further address the conundrum of thinking and/or acting wrong, one has to ask the question: what or who determines the wrong—is it not true that in someone's lexicon a "wrong" is sometimes a "right?"

For example, is there not a universal agreement that "bashing babies for sport" is a wrong, a wrong every time? We'll accept that as a universal truth, but what about bashing an oncoming baby's head, when, at the time of birth, the mother's life is in danger and/or the baby suffers from a lethal congenital disorder? The killing of a human fetus under this latter circumstance renders (in some people's minds) the wrong null and void. It is a moral conundrum of the first order—if and when a "wrong" becomes a "right?"

For whatever reason—medical or not—the human is capable of thinking and performing a wrongful act—one just knows it, because it makes one feel bad, oftentimes after the act is completed. A mother or father may have said that such an act is wrong, producing that bad feeling; a pastor or a mentor may have said what he was doing was wrong. Whatever the reason, one's conscience tells us a thought or an act is wrong. Is it not true, though, despite an active conscience, human beings are still capable, at any moment, of an evil or wrongful act?

Today, sex and sin are so intertwined that to say one may mean the same thing as saying the other. For Jackie Moreland, our chief character, and for many others, the acts of sex are a lifelong thrill, but they can be a heavy load that bears down hard on them like being caught in a fast moving waterfall. Now, after years of excessive sexual activity, Jackie has slowed down and lost some of the thrill of the conquest—just rewards, you might say, for the life that he has lived. Now, if he does get an erection, he may not sustain it or reach a climax in a marriage setting between him and his wife. However, as we shall see, he is still capable of completing the sex act in a setting of an extramarital affair between him and another woman. Now, furthermore, it is somewhat ironic that he can still fantasize about being with a woman, resulting in a successful erection and climax. No doubt, there is a psychological hang-up, a twisted touch of reality that is inexplicable. Is there a genetic makeup which is preyed upon by a society that fosters promiscuity? As always, the moment of release, whether heightened by drugs or not, stimulates the body like nothing else. But it is a momentary "high," the post-climatic fall stopped by the reality life must go on, there is work to be done, there is more life to live, and there is at least one other person to answer to in this life or another.

Let's face it, sexual addiction is basically no different from any other addiction that can ruin a person's life, even bring it to a premature ending. Living a life of extramarital sex is no different from being an alcoholic or a drug addict. The diminished heterosexual activity may be the result of a physical impairment, but the psychological scourge and the continual secret self-administered sexual acts are relentless and invariably followed by the consequences of guilt and shame. No one knows what our "hero" knows; he may have an undisclosed habit of seeking pornographic depictions on the internet that results in an erection, masturbation, and climax. It's clear the human being is a complicated animal often driven by the throes of sexual desires. And being driven by sexual desires, he or she may hurt those they love. We shall see what the human being is capable of and how he or she reacts to that capability.

To Jackie the game of baseball is not boring. You have to watch the players in the field, the batters at bat, the scoreboard that lights up the score inning by inning, the balls and strikes thrown by the pitcher, and the fans. First, he watches the pitcher to see the type of pitches he is throwing. Either pitcher often will throw an assortment of speed and off-speed pitches. Is the pitcher throwing strikes, moving the ball in and out, or up and down? Is his fastball up and are the batters putting the ball into the outfield. Second, Jackie pays attention to the location and movements of the fielders and watches how they react to a ball hit into the field of play or in foul territory. Third, he watches the movements and decisions of the umpires. Fourth, he watches the base runners who were getting signals from the first and third base coaches. And finally fifth, he watches the batter who was also getting signals from the third base coach or the dugout.

In the first game with Duke University, and all subsequent games in the series, North Carolina was the visiting team; therefore, it was logical for Jackie to sit along the first base line and just past the Carolina dugout. The usual netting did not protect the fans behind first base; therefore, he came with a glove in case a foul ball came in his direction.

The game, played in the neutral ballpark in Durham, North Carolina, the home of the minor league Bulls, would normally be played on the Duke campus. But expecting a crowd of at least five thousand, Duke University was willing to pay whatever rent was required. Since the North Carolina Tar Heels were guests of Duke and the designated visitors, they batted first.

CHAPTER TWO

"Baseball: a blooper into short right field landed softly for a single."

Jackie watched the batter swing, heard a dull crack of the bat, and saw a blooper into short right field land safely for a single. After a lazy bounce, the baseball settled still in the outfield grass—as quiet as a feather falling on a carpet. The opposing team's right fielder had no chance to catch the ball; he grabbed it by his bare hand and sent a lazy underhanded looper to the second baseman, no more than ten yards away. Jackie was relieved. It was the visiting team's first hit of the game and it ruined any chance the opposing pitcher might have thrown a no-hitter. The day was the last Friday in April; the game was the first in a three-day, three game series between the North Carolina Tar Heels and its bitter rival, the Duke University Blue Devils. Spring of that year was nearly over. The temperature that day was going into the eighties; the sun and clouds went in and out, playing a game of hide and seek. The crowd was sometimes lively and vociferous, but it barely filled half of the neutral ballpark.

Jackie Moreland, as a student at the University of North Carolina, lived on campus, studied psychology, and went to as many athletic events as he could. At all outdoor day games he attended during the baseball season, he was sensitive to the effects of the sun on his white skin; he wore a long sleeve University of North Carolina pullover to protect his arms. A five-fingered baseball glove covered most of his left hand and wrist. He'd already had at least a half dozen operations for skin cancer, the most serious of which was a melanoma-in-situ of the back—Jackie could not see it or feel it. Because of the seriousness of the diagnosis, the scar from the first excision was removed with a wide, one-to-two inch margin. The examining pathologist read the second specimen as "free of residual disease"—in other words it was a cure.

The other operations were excisions for a wide spectrum of skin lesions, all related to a lifelong exposure to the rays of the sun. In addition to the melanoma, the premalignant or malignant growths all had different names: actinic keratosis (reactive skin growth secondary to sun damage), Bowen's disease or carcinoma-in-situ, basal cell carcinoma, and squamous cell carcinoma.

Like a baseball, Jackie had the evidence of stitches all over his skin. As far as doctors and he knew, these premalignant and malignant lesions were not life threatening. However, the propensity for his skin to form these tumors was not going to change—he had played tennis since he was twelve years old and only later in life had he attempted to quell the damage the sun produced. Even a sunscreen lotion with a SPF of thirty or more could not prevent the telltale freckles that came in the spring with the first exposure to the sun. Jackie was constantly reminded that from freckles, melanomas may arise.

The day of the first Duke game, Jackie did not think he needed sunscreen; because a baseball cap, the long-sleeve pullover, and long pants covered, so he thought, all areas of exposed skin. As he was a white male with blond hair and pale skin, Jackie kept trying to hide his wrists from the sun; but the day after the game, he discovered he had been unsuccessful. The skin over the wrist and the back of his right hand was pink and blanched easily with a little manual pressure; a similar, but narrow, band of sunburn covered part of the skin over the metacarpals, the long bones in the hand between the wrist and fingers. It was clearly evident that some parts of his body did require sunscreen.

Around Jackie were fans of various stripes, young and old, who wore different shades of blue: light blue for the Carolina team and dark blue for the Duke team. In the section to his right sat under-graduate and graduate students from both schools. In his section, right behind the North Carolina dugout, there was a mixture of older adults, young families with children, and young couples of college age. The conversation around him was a mixture of casual, inane comments and technical observations on the game. The latter exchanges were quite rare.

Just after the blooper to right field that fell in for a single, four young adult Caucasian males came down the aisle and stood above Jackie hoping, he guessed, he would get up and move over. Instead, he went into the aisle and waited for them to find and take the available seats—the entire park was general admission. He knew immediately that two of them were not for Carolina; they had on dark blue baseball caps and Polo shirts, both with the big "D" stitched on them. Jackie first reaction was, "Oh shit, I sure hope they will not create any disturbance," but he decided to see if they were going to be friendly and acknowledge his existence. They all had five o'clock shadows; therefore, he knew they had just come from work. They had taken time to change clothes.

Jackie caught the eye of one sitting right next to him and said, "Hello, I'm Jackie Moreland," while he offered his right hand in friendship.

He gave Jackie a firm handshake and said, "I'm Larry Bumgardner."

"You guys must have just come from work. Have you guys been here before?" Jackie queried.

"We did. One of the guys had been here before and knew the lay of the land and where to park. The seats aren't bad for ten dollars. By your dress I can tell you are a Carolina fan. Did you graduate from Carolina?" Larry asked.

"Not yet, but I'm due to graduate next year. How about you, did you graduate from Duke?" Jackie responded.

"Frank, down there on the end, is a Duke graduate; the guys in the middle are Carolina graduates...me, I came down here from the Northeast and adopted the Blue Devils. Tell me, we're relatively new to Durham and the triangle—why is there so much animosity between the two schools?" Larry asked.

Jackie responded, "I'll give you three obvious answers: first, one school is a public state university and the other is an endowed private university, formerly Trinity College; second, the two schools, from the Atlantic Coast Conference, are only eight miles apart; and three, there has been stiff competition between the two schools since just after the turn of the century. It makes for a bitter rivalry. The hostility between the two schools has been passed down from generation to generation. It is extremely rare to find a fan that supports both schools. And, I think, before or after matriculation, the students often are as different from each other as the schools are."

"Well, that's the best explanation of many I've received. Thank you," Larry came right back to Jackie.

Jackie responded, "You're welcome. You know, it really doesn't have to be that way." "Boy, do I know," Larry said with a sigh.

Frank, the Duke fan—Carolina fans call them "Dookies"—down at the end, piped up and asked, "Larry, who's that you're talking to?" He knew Jackie was a Carolina fan; Jackie hoped he didn't want to stir up something.

Larry answered in an even, conciliatory voice, "Oddly enough, his name is Jackie Moreland and he is soon to graduate from North Carolina."

Frank came right back to Larry and said, "Larry, be careful, you know they have funny ideas, like they think public education is the best."

Jackie jumped right in and responded to the Frank in dark blue, "Frank, there is no problem. I've been vaccinated, and the shots included antiserum against a dark shade of blue." Thank goodness, several people around Jackie laughed at the exchange and went back to watching the game—no harm, no foul, except for Frank who spit out, "Asshole."

Jackie let that epitaph pass, but he couldn't let pass what happened next.

Out of the corner of his eye, he caught a glint from the sun which had hit a reflective surface. Frank had raised a small bottle to his lips, swallowed and quickly lowered his hand and hid the bottle—in a violation of the law, he had brought into the park a small bottle of liquor and was in the process of drinking from it.

"Larry," Jackie said, "tell Frank to wrap that bottle in something and pass it clown here and one of us will get rid of it. Otherwise, I'll have to call security and he'll be thrown out of the ballpark."

Larry casually went over and stood in front of Frank—there was a brief conversation. Frank sent Jackie a hard look and mouthed, "I'll get you, motherfucker!" But he proceeded to wrap the bottle in a game-day statistical sheet and hand it to Bumgardner.

Larry took the package and headed for the men's room avoiding security. He came back and told Jackie he had emptied the bottle and deposited it deep into the bin that held used paper towels. Jackie stayed in his seat, but he never felt comfortable the whole game. Frank sent him fierce looks with movements of his mouth that appeared to represent the F-word or A-word in some form or fashion—sometimes both in the same string of profanity. Jackie turned away, determined not to look at Frank for the rest of the game. He was hoping the game would get out of hand and he could leave early. That was not to happen.

Two young couples behind him were friends and he caught pieces of their animated conversation. Halfway through the game, one of the couples rose to leave. Jackie overheard part of a comment from just behind him and next to the couple leaving: "I'm sorry about your headache, but we'll be at home, come on over and well chill out and have a brew." The expression, "chill out," was a common expression from the eighties, nineties, and the first decades of the twenty-first century.

Whenever Jackie, heard, "chill out," he recalled the well-regarded movie, The Big Chill, and the sutured wrists of the body of Kevin Costner, portraying Alex. The thrust of the movie was the question of why Alex was so unhappy, why he had committed suicide, and why his friends were different, if, indeed, they were. Each of his friends had a story to tell and each had their own share of failures and successes, as is true of life. This overriding theme led to some deep philosophical discussions about the meaning of life and how each character went about living it.

One male character, for example, was a drug addict and he received the brunt of the more poignant observations. One female character, single and alone, was determined to have a baby and could see no reason why one of her male friends couldn't be the father. Another female was acutely depressed by Alex's suicide, leading to uncontrolled weeping in the shower. At one time she and Alex had been lovers. And so it went, a collage of well-educated men and women gathered to morn a dead friend, who had taken his own life. A few people, some experts and some not, call suicide "self-murder," as in you killed yourself. For some people that designation put more stigmata on the victim than was unnecessary.

To this day, the bathroom scene where they sang "Joy to the World" by Three Dog Night moved Jackie. Similarly, in the very first scene depicting Alex's funeral, one of the female actors played the haunting Credence Clearwater Revival tune, Bad Moon Rising: "Don't go around tonight, well, it's bound to take your life, there's a bad moon on the rise." That rendition of a very successful and moving song epitomized the mood of the movie and the potentially dangerous habits of the engaging cast.

This moving song always hit home for Jackie: his grandfather had taken a pistol and shot himself in the head in the fall of 1929; his death rocked Jackie's father and many others that fateful year. His grandfather, eerily similar to his father, suffered from a lifelong case of untreated clinical depression, chronic lung disease secondary to lifelong smoking, cardiac arrhythmia or atrial fibrillation, gallstones, and chronic alcoholism. Both of them finally stopped drinking, but continued smoking cigarettes. They were sedentary and overweight and decried their fellow human beings. The genes and the fateful odds were against them; his grandfather was dead at the age of 47. Fortunately, his father lived until he was 75.

CHAPTER THREE

"...some of Jackie's boyhood friends didn't play ball."

Jack Simmons, the North Carolina catcher, who sent the blooper into right field for a single, reached second base after the Duke starting pitcher balked, failing to step off the rubber, when he tried to pick Simmons off first base. Now Carolina had a man in scoring position with two outs in the bottom of the second inning and the score nothing to nothing. Jackie wasn't surprised when Duke sent their pitching coach out to confer with their starter, because this series with Duke was to have an impact on the seeding for the Atlantic Coast Conference and NCAA tournaments. The conference at the mound was one indicator of the importance of this game and the remaining two games of the series. For Duke and North Carolina, tied for second place in the conference, this series would determine the second seed for the conference tournament, which would be in a new park in Greensboro, North Carolina. Jack cooled his heels by sitting on the second base bag. After speaking with the pitcher, the catcher, and the four infielders, the Duke pitching coach went back to his perch in the home team dugout.

As best as Jackie could remember, he'd played some kind of "ball" all his life. He loved the games for the competition, camaraderie, and exercise. His neighborhood, the Dogwood Circle, had enough boys to play a full game of football, baseball and, of course, basketball. He also played tennis; but, to his regret later in life, he did not play golf at an early age. The boys, who participated in the athletic games, had to be tough, because the football and baseball games were played on the rough gravel and asphalt street that made up his neighborhood in Statesville. Basketball, played on dirt courts, was just as rough, not because of the playing surface, but because of the rugged man-to-man defense that was played. There was no one to call fouls and the boys went home bruised and battered, sometimes mad, sometimes crying, or both. That did not stop them from coming back the next day or night for more.

A total of ten boys, all about the same age—nine to twelve years old—ran around together. Usually their summer days began on bikes, but they oftentimes split up into athletic or sexual games. Luke, who lived three houses down from Jackie and his brother, was the biggest adolescent boy and he had the best build and was the best athlete. Gray, who lived between Jackie and Luke, was the best looking: dark brown curly hair and equally dark brown eyes. He, too, was a well-built, natural athlete. The third boy, Benjamin, was the smallest and quietest and lived just three houses up from Jackie and Jason. Around the circle there was Felix, who was big for his age, equally quiet, and not an athlete. Among the gang, Felix was known as a mamma's boy. He did not participate in many of these boyhood activities, except for the sexual games—that is, when he could get out of the house. Felix lived next door to Timothy who was tall and lanky with bad acne. He also had bad eyesight so he didn't play in the athletic games at all. Across the street from Felix and Timothy lived a second Benjamin and his younger brother, Nathan. These two skinny boys played in all the games and generally took the brunt of the physical trauma, often resulting in tears and a limp home.

On a warm summer day morning, when school was out, the boys of Dogwood Circle were on their bikes, riding around the oval tract. They paused after a hard ride up the left side (looking from below) of the circle. Jackie finished well ahead of the others and had time to catch his breath. He was surprised when the last of the group, the first Benjamin, shouted out breathlessly, "Jackie, Jackie, Jackie!"

Jackie was taken aback, but played along with Benjamin, "Whatie, whatie, whatie?"

"I'm glad to see you," Benjamin said, catching his breath as best he could.

"But you see me every day," Jackie responded incredulously.

"I know, but I'm still glad to see you."

"OK, Benjamin, I'm glad to see you, too."

But Benjamin was really intent on finding out if they were going to play one of their secret outdoor games and asked, "Are we going into the woods today?"

Jackie intentionally played down his response to the question in order to tease Benjamin a little, "Gosh, Benjamin, I don't know. We'll have to poll the group and see if there is a majority opinion as to whether or not we should go into the woods. You know we have never been caught, but today just might be the day we get caught, and besides, most of the boys may want to play ball."

The boys had all finally arrived and gotten off their bikes and gathered beside the road. The most vocal of the group, Gray, said, "I don't know why we can't do both."

"Yea," said Luke, "it's a summer day...I don't why we can't do both."

"Well, that settles it—there's no reason to take a poll—we can do both," Jackie concluded and added, "Those who want to play ball meet at the bottom of the circle. The others who want to go into the woods, meet in the usual place near Timothy's house. Those who decide to do both can meet up in the woods after the game."

It was an easy separation, because not all of the boys played ball—a small fringe group did not participate in sports at all. Those non-playing, predominately preadolescent males, met in secret groups for sexual games—games that were not as competitive as the ball games. However, a certain amount of camaraderie was necessary to keep these sexual games alive and interesting. Often, then, a group of six or more gathered in the woods for simultaneous masturbation. Of course, this activity was not called masturbation—the boys used the terms "circle jerk," or "jack-off," or simply "hand job." Interestingly enough, some of the young boys watched only their on hand and penis, while others watched everybody else but themselves. The boy who "came" first garnered boos and laughter, while the one who lasted the longest before coming was designated the ringleader for the day and could call the shots, so to speak. As an aside, it was highly unusual for any of the boys to masturbate a second time any one day.

To Jackie, as he remembered it, this activity was all well and good as far it went—circle jerks among kids this age would not be considered abnormal. However, there was a smaller group of boys who "advanced" to jacking off another member of the group. Certainly, that might suggest some degree of sexual deviancy, but at that age it was unlikely to be a characteristic that would extend into adolescence or adulthood.

Now, things didn't always stop there for some of the gang. Timothy and Jackie went one step further: they began to meet apart from the group and perform "blowjobs" (the technical term would be fellatio) on each other. Blowjobs were satisfying to the point of ejaculation, but, no doubt Jackie felt it was an homosexual act and he always felt ashamed after it was over. Therefore, it was no surprise that Jackie had to go first, because he could not perform the act right after he had "come." Furthermore, Timothy and he, again in secret apart from the other boys, would periodically meet in Timothy's garage apartment for what is best described as "dry intercourse"—naked they would hump each other until ejaculation occurred, sometimes simultaneously. Out of the moment, there was heavy guilt for Jackie and the realization that what he had just done something that was abnormal and wrong. That all stopped when Timothy went off to private school, and Jackie never did seek or find any other boy that he would go that far with. The height of the thrill and the depth of the guilt counteracted each other. Fate or not, Jackie never let a relationship with a boy go that far, but he never ceased to wonder if he was to have gay tendencies the rest of his life. This side of Jackie's life was counterbalanced by his lust for the opposite sex. He always wondered if his hormones were out-of-balance one way or the other—which is to wonder if he could go both ways.

We, then, go back to the group who didn't play ball, but who did meet in the woods for sexual games. In addition to round-robin masturbation, this group occasionally met with one preadolescent girl who was willing to take off her underpants, and let the boys see her vagina. Interestingly enough, considering how far they had come with mutual jackoffs, the showing the girl gave never got to the "playing doctor stage," when one of the boys would "examine" her female sexual parts.

No doubt the boys fantasized and talked about getting to the playing doctor stage, but that just got them in the mood to jackoff. There is little doubt that the thoughts of sex occupied the group's preadolescent and adolescent minds, day and night. It was evident, and certainly normal, that all of these boys would become law-abiding and well-adjusted adults. How many would reflect back on their preadolescent and adolescent days? There might be times when they remembered their days of boyhood sex, but they certainly didn't allow any of those memories to affect their adulthood years. For them it was a growing phase and a basis for understanding their subsequent serious relationships with the opposite sex.

CHAPTER FOUR

"...but you know what I think, I think that some of the girls did it on purpose."

With Simmons on second base and two outs in the Carolina second inning, the fourth batter in the rotation, hitting from the left side, sent a sharp line drive into right field, driving Simmons home for the first run of the game. The crowd in light blue gave Simmons and his mate a standing ovation—the standing part was unusual for a RBI single, but it was indicative of the intensity of the rivalry and the importance of the game. The next batter in the inning sent a grounder to second base that was easily relayed to first base for the final out in that inning. After the first two innings the score was: UNC 1, Duke 0.

Even later in life, it was easy for Jackie Moreland to picture the predominately rural region of western North Carolina: verdant, rolling hills dotted with small communities and broken by ribbons of concrete and asphalt. Interstate 40, shaped like a parabola, went from Wilmington in the east to Murphy in the west and then onto the west coast; serpentine Interstate 85 went from Petersburg, Virginia, through the South Carolina border below Charlotte, the queen city. I-85 ended in Montgomery, Alabama. The piedmont triad of Winston-Salem, Greensboro and High Point was the jumping off point for the gentle rise of land that made up the western part of the state.

As we have noted, Jackie and his brother and sisters were born and raised in Statesville, North Carolina; less than halfway between the piedmont and mountain regions of the state. Outside his relationships with his siblings, his earliest childhood memories, as we have noted, consisted of a mixture of events in school, playing sports and games, and riding bikes. The latter had the potential for accidents and the school experiences, as it turned out, had potential for controversy.

The boys didn't think about the risks for either, and it was probably just as well. But if they did think about it, riding bikes always had the potential for a wreck: bump the curb, hit a car, lose control, and hit the rugged surface of the street were all possibilities for an accident. But, in Jackie's memory, the worse mishap occurred as he was riding on the handlebars of Luke's bike, when they were coming down the entrance to their neighborhood. For some reason, which Jackie didn't recall and couldn't surmise, the hill was not paved and it was steep enough that coming down, they could obtain considerable speed. Thus, they were going too fast and about two-thirds of the way down the hill, Jackie got his foot caught in the front wheel and it locked, flipping the bike over and scattering the bike and riders all over the graveled hill. Jackie didn't know how, and could not surmise how they suffered only bruises and lacerations. The wreck scared the boys and they relived the accident, wondering how they could have survived it. No doubt both of them got a "tongue-lashing" or worse.

Jackie's memory of an incident early in his life was of an entirely different matter and one that he would dwell on and regret the rest of his life. He and a small group of boys and girls, age's five to seven, went to a neighborhood kindergarten. Indoors they played games, built houses with blocks, and listened to the daily stories read by their teacher. Outdoors they played in a sandbox or swung on swings. When the teacher wasn't outside, and when they were certain she was not looking, they also climbed trees. Those few occasions, when one of the kids fell out of a tree, were kept secret and the victim just had to "suck it up."

The kindergarten was in the basement of the teacher's home and a steep set of stairs came down from the floor above. The boys and girls never went to the floor above, but sometimes some of them would sit on the stairs during frequent breaks. Now, in the nineteen fifties and sixties, the girls often wore dresses and the boys, long khaki pants. So, when the girls would sit on the steps, the boys would try to look up their dresses and see if they could see their panties. More times than not, some of the boys would be successful in seeing one of the girl's underwear, which you could imagine was white.

Cindy was a perceptive, bright and attractive six year-old girl in her first year of organized school. But, of all the girls there, Cindy was the one who was open to and relished the boys' attention. Well into the fall term, Cindy noticed Jackie looking up her dress and, in a loud, strident voice, called him on it, "Jackie, stop looking up my dress!" (Jackie didn't express his opinion then, but it was clear to him that Cindy was "cutting off her nose to spite her face.")

The teacher, Mrs. Overton, had just started down the stairs when she heard Cindy's declaration. She immediately cleared the stairs and asked Jackie to come up into her den for a lithe talk. She started with a question, "Were you looking up Cindy's dress?"

"Well, yes I was, but it wasn't like I was looking up her dress on purpose," he answered, demurely. He lied, the beginning of a life-long habit of "misrepresenting the facts."

"And, I imagine all the boys have done what you did, yet they don't do it on purpose," she responded knowingly.

"Yes, Ma'me."

"Jackie, I don't care how many boys do it, it is unacceptable behavior and show disrespect for the girls. Whatever thrill you get out of it can easily become a habit and stay with you the rest of your life," she surmised, laying her hand on his shoulder—both her voice and her hand were heavy on his young soul.

"I'm sorry, Mrs. Overton, but you know what I think, I think some of the girls sit on the stairs on purpose, daring the boys to have a look up their dress," he said, rather forthrightly.

"Well, on purpose or not, you can rest assured that this will not happen again," she said with conviction and added, "you go home for the rest of the day and you tell your mother what happened here."

She showed him to the door and went back down stairs and announced to the class that from now on, there'll be no sitting on the steps. The boys didn't boo, but they wanted to; a few girls giggled, hands over their mouths.

Jackie told his mom what had happed and said he wouldn't do it anymore—which was another lie. He never stopped looking up girls' and women's dresses whenever the opportunity presented itself. It was just another manifestation of the fact that for him, women were sexual objects. And, for Jackie, it was already an ingrained habit by age seven. Seeing women as sexual objects is a curse for many, if not most, men and sadly, no amount of individual or group therapy can overcome it.

CHAPTER FIVE

"...nice eye candy..."

The third inning came and went in a hurry. Except far a double into the left field corner by the Duke Centerfielder, neither side produced a base runner—the one runner for Duke was stranded. The crowd was quiet; yet they were restless. Jackie was amazed at the number of young women wearing tank tops and short shorts, displaying smooth, even tans, in April for God's sake. No question for Jackie, but they were nice "eye candy." The score remained UNC 1, Duke 0.

As I have said, Jackie grew up on Dogwood Circle in Statesville, North Carolina. Actually it wasn't a circle, but it was really an oval, an upside and a downside flanked by two hills. Except for the top entrance, the "circle" was paved with rough asphalt imbedded with small pebbles. The surface, you might imagine, made the games the boys played on the street rough and fraught with the likelihood of injury—no doubt they were prey to scrapes and bruises during both the seasons of football and baseball. Jackie simply considered the scrapes and bruises part of the game—he pressed on with no thought for tomorrow or, the next day, for that matter.

How about siblings? Did Jackie have brothers and sisters? One brother was named Jason; the name derived from the Greek word for "healer." It's an appropriate name since he would eventually become a doctor. Jackie had two twin sisters, Beatrice and Bobbie. In age the girls were in the middle between the two boys. Jackie, Jason, Bea, and Bobbie were athletic and competitive—loving, but, in the moment, extremely intense and unyielding.

The family name was Moreland and the father was a doctor. He had married a nurse he met in medical school and, incredibly, her name was Jacqueline. It was decided early on that she would retain the longer name, but she could never stopped reacting and answering to "Jackie."

As time went by, the marriage between Frank, the father, and Jacqueline, the mother, developed disruptive seams that would never heal—Frank Moreland was a functioning alcoholic and his wife was an enabler. Bad karma went along with numerous arguments. The children did their best to stay away and avoid the combatants. The psychological and emotional stress experienced by the family caused a great deal of "acting out" by the kids. Slowly, all members of the family showed signs of depression and anxiety. All, but Frank, at one time or another, required counseling. As Jackie had noted with his grandfather, his father had multiple medical problems and, besides alcoholism, suffered from a moderate case of clinical depression.

CHAPTER SIX

"...oh, God, I've got another splitting headache."

In the bottom of the fourth inning Duke tied the score, one to one. The leadoff batter worked the count to three balls and two strikes. Much to the chagrin of the Carolina coach, the umpire called the next pitch a ball and Duke had a runner on first base. It was no surprise to anyone in the ballpark when the runner stole second base. Now there was a man on second with nobody out. The third base coach, when the count got to two balls and a strike on the next batter, called a bunt to sacrifice the runner to third base where a hit, a ground ball to the right side, or a long fly to the outfield would bring the runner in from third base. The play was executed to perfection and the man on second easily made it to third. There was only one out when the next batter sent a high ball to centerfield, sending the man home from third, tying the score at one to one after the fourth inning.

The Moreland family had a mutt named "Socks," because the dog was black with four white feet. She was a happy mongrel that liked to chase squirrels and run after thrown rocks or sticks. In the house at night, Socks was subdued and quiet unless someone came to the door—then she let out a howl.

Practically speaking, the kids could not remember when their dog wasn't part of the family. In particular, Jackie and Jason argued over whom the dog belonged to. Looking back, it seemed extremely silly, but the boys decided they would have to cut the dog in half so that both of them could have at least part of the dog. Of course, the argument became deadlocked when they could not decide how to cut the animal in two. The twins laughed to the point of hysterics, when it became apparent that the boys could not solve the silly conundrum.

"You boys are so silly, even to the point of being ridiculous," Bea said with a bit of sarcasm.

"Well, he's not your dog, so you have no say so in this whatsoever," Jason responded, emphatically.

It was the month of June and all four kids were out in the yard playing with Socks. Their mother came out in the yard with a reminder: "I know you are on vacation, but that doesn't mean you don't have responsibilities. I have asked you to clean up your rooms and make your beds...oh, God, I've got another splitting headache."

Bea responded to her mother, "Mom, you have got to go see a doctor. These headaches are too severe and come on too often."

"I know, you're right. I'll get an appointment as soon as possible," her mother acquiesced.

Jacqueline finished the breakfast dishes, made an appointment with the family doctor and went straight to bed—it wasn't a migraine, but it was as bad as she could remember. She darkened the room and covered her eyes. Jacqueline hadn't mentioned it to anybody, but what really scared her was the fact that she was losing control of her left arm—from time to time it got so bad she couldn't use the arm at all. She had always been in good health, was an active tennis player, and often ran the "circle" to stay in shape. Frank stayed home that day, aware of Jacqueline's headaches; but, until then, he wasn't aware of the trouble with her left arm. He knew then that his wife had a major problem in her head, and she needed to have a MRI scan to rule out a brain tumor. He hoped that the fact she hadn't had a seizure was a good sign—maybe the tumor was not large and was in a location amenable to surgical removal.

The next day Frank made an appointment for Jacqueline to be seen by a neurosurgeon that practiced in Statesville and had an appointment at the North Carolina Hospitals in Chapel Hill. Dr. Simmons had a good reputation and decades of experience—he was known for his surgical expertise. He was able to see Jacqueline within a few days of her latest headache.

"Dr. Simmons, thank you for seeing us so quickly," Frank said, relief in his voice.

"No problem, your wife needed to be seen as soon as possible." Directing his questions to Jacqueline, Dr. Simmons asked, "Now, before I examine you, Mrs. Moreland, tell me how long this problem has been going on?"

She responded to his question, "I think the headaches have been occurring nearly every day for about six weeks."

"Describe the headaches for me," he instructed her in a soft, but commanding voice.

"By the afternoon of most every day, the headache is severe, and although it is worse on the right side, it seemed as if it involves my whole head."

"Where do they start?" he asked.

"Just above my right eye," she answered without hesitation.

"Do the headaches pound or pulsate?" he continued with the questions.

"No, they are constant and just hurt enough to put me to bed in a dark room," she answered.

"Does the rest in the dark room alleviate the headaches?" he asked again.

"Somewhat, but they never go away," she answered, her eyes misting.

"Do the headaches respond to analgesics?" he continued.

"What do you mean by analgesics?" she asked, thinking he must be talking about aspirin.

"Over-the-counter pain relievers," he explained.

"I try taking Advil, but I have no complete relief unless I am able to sleep, which doesn't happen very often."

Dr. Simmons paused, thinking, a crease down his forehead. Jacqueline didn't like his expression—she was fearful the news was not going to be good—and, as a matter of fact, because of the weakness in her left arm, down deep she knew the news wasn't going to be good. But there had to be an x-ray, so she was not quite ready to panic.

He spoke up after a few pregnant moments and asked, "Is there anything else that's been bothering you?"

"Yes, I have weakness in my left arm," she admitted, knowing that would probably tip the scales of what, up to that point in time, could have been any number of explanations for her symptoms.

"Well, tell me, have you lost normal function in that arm?" he asked, knowing that would be a critical sign.

"At first, it was just weakness, but it has been progressively worse and I began to lose the ability to use it all," she explained, her voice weak and low.

"I missed that. Did you say you weren't able to move it?"

"Right," she virtually whispered.

Mrs. Morehead, I'll not mince words with you: what you have described to me suggests there is something going on in the right side of your head that would explain these signs and symptoms. Now, the only way to be sure of that would be to perform what is called an MRI, initials for "Magnetic Resonance Imagining," an x-ray of your head and brain, usually following a pre-injection of contrast material. Do you know if you are allergic to contrast material?"

"No, I have no known allergies." Jacqueline broke up and cupped her head in her hands. She looked up and stammered, "When I lost the normal function of my left arm, I knew it was something serious."

Dr. Simmons replied, "Look, right now we can't be sure of anything. If the x-ray shows a mass, it is still possible it is a benign process, like a meningioma. If we explore your brain and find a mass, the only way we can be sure of the diagnosis is to take a biopsy and have that tissue examined by a pathologist. Do you follow me so far?"

"Yes," she said demurely.

"OK, let's not get ahead of ourselves; we have to set you up for a MRI."

The MRI confirmed a right cerebral mass the size of a golf ball located near the motor strip that controlled muscular function on the left side of the body. Surgery was scheduled for the following day: using burr holes and a bone saw, a bone flap was raised on the right side just above the tumor. Dr. Simmons easily removed the mass which was determined to be an astrocytoma, a grade two to three malignant tumor of brain origin. Jacqueline came through the surgery with only a temporary paralysis of the left side of the body. He was able to take a rim of normal brain tissue without risking her with permanent paralysis. She was expected to make a full recovery and was scheduled to start rehabilitation the week after surgery. Dr. Simmons and the oncology team determined it was necessary to add irradiation, but not chemotherapy, to the treatment plan.

Frank and the kids were by her side throughout her surgery, immediate recovery and rehabilitation. She was given medicine for her pain and headaches, but both rapidly resolved. Dr. Simmons tried to make it clear that they were not quite out of the woods yet, but he was confident that in five years' time she would be cured. He didn't say, but he knew a five year cure with less than a four-grade tumor with irradiation could be expected. Particularly, in Jackie's mother's case, considering how easy it was to remove the entire tumor and how the rest of the brain looked, he had an unusual amount of optimism. It turns out his optimism was justified.

Chapter Seven

"A dare, Jackie? You should be ashamed of yourself."

Neither Duke nor Carolina scored in the fifth through the seventh inning. There were double plays on both sides that ended each half of the inning. The score remained one to one. The crowd sang "Take Me Out to the Ballgame," as they stood for the seventh inning stretch. The sky had turned grey from the thickening of the clouds, but the expected showers held off for the duration of the game.

Mrs. Walton was Jackie's third-grade teacher, and a great teacher she was. She was large, very large, but as warm as she was large. One day Jackie raised his hand to speak and Mrs. Walton recognized him, "Yes, Jackie Moreland."

"Mrs. Walton, I have a poem that I would like to recite to the class."

"By all means, we would love to hear you recite some poetry," his teacher responded with enthusiasm.

"Christopher Columbus sailed the ocean blue, hit a rock and pissed all over the crew!"

No one moved, no one spoke, but there was an audible gasp from many members of the class. It must have been that some didn't understand the rhyme or were too stunned to react in any way.

"Jackie, that is totally unacceptable. Don't you realize how dirty what you call a poem, sounds?" Mrs. Walton, red in the face, responded with vehemence.

She added, "Class, please read today's lesson while I take Jackie to the principal's office."

Sterling Wilder was a teacher for twenty years before he became a principal. Mrs. Walton was one of his favorite teachers; he held her in very high regard and trusted her judgment explicitly.

"Mrs. Walton, who do you have in tow there?" he asked, when she and Jackie were shown into the office.

"Jackie Moreland, Mr. Wilder," Mrs. Walton said with a tone of regret.

"What has he done that you feel like he should see me right away?" he asked.

"He recited a dirty poem in front of the class just now," she responded and added, "It contained the word, 'pissed'."

Mr. Wilder stepped in front of Jackie and asked, "Jackie Moreland, what in the world were you thinking?" He then added, "Jackie this is totally out of character for you. You know we can't let that behavior go by without punishment."

Jackie paused. The silence was so palpable it was deafening! "Mr. Wilder, I don't know what came over me. It all started on the playground. Several of the boys were repeating this rhyme and one, talking to me, said, "I'll bet you won't repeat it in class."

Mr. Wilder hit the intercom button and said, "Mrs. Johnson, please get Dr. or Mrs. Moreland on the line please."

"Mr. Wilder, Mrs. Moreland's on line one," Mrs. Johnson announced.

The principal punched in line one and said, "Mrs. Moreland, can you come to my office right away. We have a disciplinary decision to make regarding your son, Jackie."

Mrs. Moreland responded, "Mr. Wilder, what has my son done?"

"He recited a dirty poem in Mrs. Walton 's class this morning," the principal answered.

"Oh, my God, that's not like Jackie—at least not the Jackie I know—I'll be there in ten minutes," Mrs. Moreland said and closed the line.

Jackie's mother was in the principal's office in ten minutes. Mr. Wilder rose and said to her, "Thank you for coming in, Mrs. Moreland. I believe you know Mrs. Walton."

"Yes, I do. Mrs. Walton, I am so very sorry that Jackie has disrupted your class in this way. This is highly unusual for Jackie, who, I believe has not been taken to the principal's office before. What was the poem? Can it be repeated?" Mrs. Moreland sighed and looked at Mr. Wilder.

"I wish I didn't have to repeat it to you, but I think it is serious enough that I don't have a choice. Fortunately, it is very short and there is only one bad word: "Christopher Columbus sailed the ocean blue, (he) hit a rock, and pissed all over the crew.'"

"Well, I am shocked, completely shocked. Jackie, look at me. What obsessed you to do such a thing and to do it in Mrs. Walton's class? To my knowledge, you have never said that word at home!"

"Mom, I'm very, very sorry that this has happened and that you had to hear it repeated. It was all a dare from one of my friends on the playground."

"A dare, Jackie? I'm so ashamed of you! Yes, you should look down!" she said emphatically.

"Mrs. Moreland, I will have to suspend Jackie for the rest of the week," Mr. Wilder interjected.

"I understand perfectly, Mr. Wilder, and I can assure you nothing like this will ever happen again. (Subsequent "acting out" events, that were not so serious, occurred, but, somehow Jackie stayed out of the principal's office.)

"Jackie, get your books. Mrs. Walton, can you give him the lessons for the rest of the week?" his mother said, great sadness and regret in her voice.

CHAPTER EIGHT

Holden Caulfield: "...I know that's all I would really want to be."

In the top of the eighth inning, Jack Simmons, the Carolina catcher, who started the second inning with a single and eventually scored, hit a home run over the right field wall with two out and the bases empty. The game went into the bottom of the eighth inning with the score Carolina 2, Duke 1.

Mrs. White taught the eighth grade, the first year at Statesville High School. Jackie Moreland was in her class and was a model student—yet, at age fourteen, his hormones were raging. He lusted after Mrs. White and fanaticized about her teaching him how adults perform sex. She was young and extremely attractive, just a few years out of college. (You can imagine that Mrs. White would have absolutely no idea that one of her students was fanaticizing about having sex with her.) Jackie couldn't have cared less that she had married a young man fresh out of college. Although he had trouble paying attention in class, it did not prevent him from being an "A" student. Frequently, he spoke up in class when Mrs. White asked a question—particularly when the question related to human relationships. Again, it was lost on Mrs. White that he was eager to answer her questions; not because he was an excellent student, but because he lusted after her in the worst way. Fortunately, Jackie never got beyond the fanaticizing stage in his sexual illusions concerning his eighth grade teacher. No doubt he was glad he wore tight underwear to class; it kept down the ever present erection and subsequent wetness .

Three years later, Jackie's class was reading "Catcher in the Rye," a novel by J. D. Salinger. Jackie readily identified with the chief character and narrator, Holden Caulfield. The following is a paper Jackie wrote after reading the book:

Depending on how you read and interpret the book, "Catcher in the Rye," any subsequent analysis of Salinger's work would conclude that it was either a complicated book or a simple, straightforward writing. I favor the latter—interpretation is easier that way. The message of the book is pretty clear: a boy in his teenage years is trying very hard to be a real person in the face of what he describes as depression, angst, and raging sex hormones. As we noted above, the story is told completely in the voice of the teenager—he is the principal protagonist. Caulfield gives us an array of inner thoughts and describes his relationships with a whole host of characters; from family members to roommates, teachers, and strangers.

He frequently and consistently tells lies. Why? For one thing it makes him see himself as mysterious; for another it makes him feel superior—sort of a "gotcha," as in, only I know what the truth is. Thus, you know he doesn't have to own up to who he is and what he is about, if anything. He rants and raves about phony people and places that come into his gestalt. Does he realize that through his many falsehoods, he is just as phony as those persons and places he describes? I doubt not. He admits he is immature, but, for a teenager, he acts and does things any older person would do.

If there is any significance to his name, Holden Caulfield, the reader is not made aware of it. He smokes incessantly and suffers from the habit, inhaling deeply. But you readily know that is part of feeling grownup and part of his rebellious nature. He has to be careful that he doesn't run out of money to buy cigarettes. We get the impression that on frequent occasions-when he has enough money—he gets drunk, an action that makes him feel worse and more depressed.

He is constantly referring to feeling sad: a so-in-so person or place or situation makes him depressed—through the story, we readily sense he is not happy, just a sad sack. Holden, through word or inference, makes us realize he is a lonely boy. Thus, in an immediate reaction we raise the question: just how much does his lack of consistent and rewarding relationships make him feel alone? Frequently, he finds himself in the late hours of the day, usually drunk, with no place to go and no companions to be with. The reader gets the feeling that if he doesn't get ahold of himself, he will die at a young age, destitute and alone, only himself to blame.

Although we know he is intelligent and has read some enlightening books, he is a poor student; for in the last bout with the books in a pricy and private school, he has flunked four of five classes. He avoided going to class or doing his assignments. If he did go to class, he was reluctant to speak up when the opportunity presented itself. He does have interesting relationships with select teachers, but they all reproach him for his laziness and inability to stay the course, do the homework and speak up in class. Holden has been kicked out of school, but he does not go straight home. Instead he gets a room in a sleazy New York hotel, avoiding his parents, but recognizing that they will know of his suspension before he gets home. He plans it that way, thinking maybe they will have had time to let the news seep in.

What are his relationships with his fellow students, his roommates? They are rather complicated and often contentious. He'll wake a roommate or someone in his dorm for no particular reason or as some kind of joke. He constantly and consistently looks on his world and relationships as opportunities to play a joke or to simply get a reaction. He shows a temper when he gets into a fight with someone who is bigger and stronger.

The only meaningful and deep relationship he has is with his younger sister, Phoebe. She adores him and brings out sincere feelings from him. It is evident that he has done things for her in the past, which personify his deep affection for her. She is smart and exhibits a self-affirming curiosity. Unfortunately, Holden is a poor example, but she doesn't see it. Phoebe decides to leave school and go anywhere with him—she even packs a bag. Finally Holden puts his foot down and makes Phoebe go back to class, telling her he has decided not to run away.

One item, one last characteristic of Holden, is his incessant use of profane language. Phoebe tells him repeatedly to stop cussing, but it is to no avail. Why does he cuss so much? The whole world is a "goddamn" this and a "goddamn" that. Everything is a seven-letter epitaph relating to something or someone that causes him angst.

Holden is a virgin—maybe he has experienced a few close calls, but there is nothing definitive. He says he doesn't understand sex; it baffles him! From time to time he may be aroused by somebody of the opposite sex, but, even with a prostitute, he cannot control his opposite reaction. It stops him and he cannot finish the act. Why is it that way? He doesn't know; he recognizes the raging hormones within, but they baffle him and he stops short of a climax. It is like his sexuality is a force from somewhere that, when it manifests itself, it seems to be alien.

What is Holden Caulfield's future? He doesn't know and neither do we. He admits he gets sick when he got home—certainly not surprising, considering his lifestyle. He will go to another school in the fall, but will he apply himself? He doesn't know; he hadn't got there yet. We are not told what kind of school it is. He asks how can you know whether or not you will apply yourself until you get there. In the final analysis he misses everybody "he told about" even that "goddamn Maurice."

Holden says, "Don't ever tell anybody anything. If you do, you start missing everybody." You get the impression that he will turn things around—potentially he is a good person, but a good person who knows not the truth.

Where does the title of the book come from? In the latter third of the book Holden tells us the title comes from a poem by Robert

Burns: "If a body meets a body coming through the rye." Holden says "...I keep picturing all these little kids playing some game in this big field of rye and all. Thousands of little kids and nobody's around—nobody big I mean—except me. And I'm standing on the edge of some crazy cliff. What I have to do, I have to catch everybody if they start to go over the cliff-I mean if they're running and they don't look where they're going, I have to come out from somewhere and catch them. That's all I do all day. I'd just me the catcher in the rye and all. I know it's crazy, but that's the only thing I'd really like to be."

In the reading of where the title of the book comes from, one sees behind his fantasy his relationship with his sister. Her, you know, he would always care for and look after, even if he has to go over the cliff to save her.

Is there any similarity between Holden Caulfield and Jackie Moreland? For one thing, we have to acknowledge the fact that we know more about Holden than we do about Jackie. But one thing is clear: both of them have made and will make mistakes—after all, they are human. The other shared characteristic is that both of them have a problem with sex, but, in detail, their problems are different. As time goes by, will they become more confident in their physical relationships with women? We can only guess that, yes, they would become more confident and mature and finally lose their virginity. In a time snapshot, we see that Jackie is a better student, even making all "A's" at some point. Finally, they both have a period when they run away from reality, acting out before maturity sets in. Jackie faces physical death; Holden faces loneliness, a death of the soul.

CHAPTER NINE

"Jackie was a unanimous selection as the biggest flirt!"

And in the bottom of the eighth inning, the first batter in the Duke lineup hit a ball over the left field fence to tie the score at two to two. The next two batters were out after hitting ground balls to the Carolina shortstop. Both teams, by the eighth inning, had replaced their starting pitcher with their late reliever or "closer" as they are called. The weather, though cloudy, continued to cooperate with no measurable precipitation. The crowd remained at about five thousand, the majority of the fans behind each dugout. Many in the crowd anticipated an extra inning affair and they were not to be denied.

We continue to hear of Jackie Moreland's exploits. in the seventh grade at one of the Statesville elementary schools, just before his matriculation to the eighth grade, the seniors worked on a class annual and took a vote for the "best" and "brightest" students in the class. It was likely to carry over into the next grade at Statesville High School. Jackie was a unanimous selection as the "biggest flirt." He was just attracted to members of the opposite sex—he dated the best looking girl in the seventh grade. Her name was Sandra, shortened to Sandy. She was a fair-skinned brunette with exquisite, delicate facial features and small body build—she had yet to completely fill out. Jackie had no direct evidence, but he surmised that her breasts were so small she didn't wear a bra.

It was in September of that final year that Beverly, one of the most popular girls in the school, started a regular dance Saturday nights after each of the Friday home games in football.

"Sandy, are you going to the dance Saturday night?" Jackie, standing close to Sandy, said with twinkling eyes, a hand on her free arm. He was tall for his age and had light hair and expressive hazel eyes, which on occasion were said to be green. He too was slim with small bones.

"Oh, yea, I'm going," Sandy responded, knowing that there would be dancing all evening until close to eleven o'clock.

"Well, do you want my mother and me to pick you up?" Jackie asked.

"No, I'm going with a bunch of girls, but you can be my date," Sandy intoned, expressing herself easily, as she was comfortable and confident with Jackie. They had been going steady since the year before this one. She was even wearing a ring.

At Beverly's home the lights in the living room were set low, making the room essentially dark. The music was conducive to slow dancing. The couples paired off and stacked out a small corner where they held each other closely and went round and round and round. Before the first song was through, Jackie felt an erection. With purpose he had worn tight fitting jockey shorts. He and Sandy, as before on many similar occasions, went pelvis to pelvis. It felt good and he knew that she knew what the score was.

Around ten-thirty, the lights went up, the music went faster, and everybody did the jitterbug or the shag—mothers and fathers on their way. All-in-all it was a good night; everybody was happy, knowing there were more dances to come—that is, as long as the couples remained an "item." Jackie obsessed about going further, determined to get a feel.

It was just the beginning of a journey that would take Jackie further and further into the clutches of an obsession with sex, heterosexual sex. But, sadly, it wasn't to be with Sandy. By the ninth grade Sandy was going steady with a football player. Jackie began to seek out less popular girls and was determined to go as far as these girls would go with him. A good example of how his modus operandi had changed occurred at the first football game after he and Sandy had broken up. He took a much less attractive girl into the trees that surrounded the stadium. There he got a feel. Things had changed and, as it turned out, not for the better. He became a rogue hunter, starting a life-long habit of chasing available, oftentimes vulnerable, girls and later fully mature women. He experienced the thrill of the chase that was missing in his earlier relationships. He fantasized about sex with all sorts of the opposite sex; he had moved on from his autoerotic relationship with his male friend, Timothy.

CHAPTER TEN

"...maybe, just maybe, he would have stayed close to home,
warmed by the relationship that started so very young in his life."

A s expected the game went into extra innings, the score remaining two to two. In the tenth inning, Carolina threatened to score; after a ground ball went into the right field for a single and the runner stole second base, the next Carolina batter struck out. The pitcher kept the man on second base with frequent steps off the rubber and faints at the bag. With the full count of three balls and two strikes, the pitcher finally picked the runner off second base. The threat to score ended and the game went into the eleventh inning. The crowd grew restless—nobody had scored since the eighth inning.

Jackie Moreland finally "scored" in the fourth year of high school. Of all places, the relationship with Catherine started in the First Presbyterian Church of Statesville. Leaders of the youth fellowship, they were frequently thrown together. In the spring of his senior year and her junior year, they both were sent to a Presbyterian youth convention in Louisville, Kentucky. Though they were not allowed to be alone in the same room, they drew close to one another, "sparked" together when they could.

Physically, they were opposites: Jackie was tall and Catherine was short. But that physical difference was in no way a problem; they both let their feelings show and it wasn't long before it became evident they were experiencing a strong sexual attraction—Jackie could not keep his hands off of Catherine and she responded in kind. By the time they got home, they were an "item" and they began to go steady.

Jackie had his driving license and the 1948 Chevrolet he drove had no central console, so Catherine was able to sit close and keep her hands free to touch sensitive areas of his body.

Frequently after their dates, Jackie parked near Catherine's house and they embraced and kissed passionately. It was a "French" kiss and neither of them could remember how that started, but it was a fore-taste of what was to come. Her skirt came up and his pants came down. There was no need to say they both lost their virginity. Right then they started a pattern of making love without a condom, but then that was early in the emphasis on protection. Somehow she didn't be-come pregnant, but that wasn't talked about—it fell on Catherine to keep the sexual activity away from the middle of her periods.

They went together for two years before Jackie went off to col-lege at the University of North Carolina at Chapel Hill. That turned out to be the breaking point in their relationship. Catherine wanted to get married, but Jackie couldn't or wouldn't do it. He was on track to do graduate work in psychology and couldn't see any way they could afford to get married. She was crushed, but somehow went on with her life, working in Christian education and eventually getting married and raising a family. For the remainder of his life, Jackie won-dered how getting married as a freshman would have turned out—maybe, just maybe, he would have stayed close to home, warmed by the relationship that started so very young in his life.

CHAPTER ELEVEN

"...he was an unhappy sot."

The baseball game went into the shank of the evening; the multiple banks of lights were turned on. Some in the crowd got up and went home. The pitchers continued to keep the other team's batters to no more than walks or in-field singles. Neither team could get anyone past second base—the remaining crowd was quite subdued. The game went into the fifteenth inning.

In Statesville, the Moreland's lived in a modest white two story, two bedroom house—the attic was turned into a third bedroom for the twin girls. The main problem with that setup was that there was no bathroom on the second floor. So Bea and Bobbie simply were the first to use the small downstairs bathroom during the school months—otherwise it was catch as catch can, every family member for himself or herself all the other months. Jacqueline, the mother, did the cooking, and breakfast was always ready by seven o'clock in the morning. That left plenty of time for the kids to catch a ride to school. Dr. Moreland had the same breakfast day in and day out: a poached egg with bacon, toast, and coffee. He commanded the table from the near end with a sternness that kept the kids on edge and their mother nervous.

"You kids got your homework done for classes today?" he bellowed out, as the twins and their brothers came to the table.

In unison they responded to their father, "Yes, sir."

Jacqueline and the children stepped lightly around Dr. Moreland, in constant fear that he would break out into one of his "tantrums." Actually, though, it was fairly peaceful in the morning—that, of course, depended on whether father had gotten drunk the night before. Either way, he was an unhappy sot, who always came home in a sour mood. Often, at that time, sparks would fly, because Jacqueline would invariably challenge him for some reason or another. The confrontation was predictable, particularly when the subject of money or his relationship with his nurse came up.

Dr. Moreland was in solo practice, specializing in diseases of the chest, a subset of internal medicine. Blanch was his one and only nurse and they had a close relationship that went back to the nineteen forties. His wife had known about their affair for years and as time went by she stopped broaching the subject—it would just cause a fight. She adjusted to the situation, planning on a divorce when the kids were out of the house. Of course, that didn't quell the bitterness that ate at her like a cancer. As a result of this constant bickering, she stayed depressed, lost weight, and did little to make herself more attractive. Were it not for her writing ability, she would have wasted away to nothing long ago. And there was something in her that allowed her to welcome each and every day, especially for the kids. Dr. Moreland, on the other hand, didn't seem to notice her waning, nor did he care. Somebody, somewhere along the way, decided he was narcissistic. There was no chance that that would be challenged or used as a reason for psychotherapy—he resisted that without so much as a discussion.

One morning Mrs. Moreland started in on her husband, "I didn't hear you come to bed. Did you drink too much last night?"

"Oh, I only had a couple," he answered her.

"Daddy," Bee interjected.

"What?" he growled.

"You had more than a couple," she added.

"You didn't see me drinking last night," he said, innocently.

"I didn't have to see you drinking," Bee said, not one to shrink from the obvious truth.

"All right, lady, I had a few, but you couldn't have known it," her father added with some prideful hurt.

"What do you mean, I couldn't have known it? I've only known that you've drunk to excess for at least ten years. All I have to do is see you stumble around and know you've had way too many," Bee expounded, gulping down her breakfast.

"All right, you two," her mother broke in and added, "this is an old saw and I'm tired of hearing about it. Neither of you is going to give in and acknowledge the truth of what the other is saying. But, no doubt, none of us would trust the words of a man who is trying to defend himself when he is in the fog of excessive alcohol."

"Well, mother, if you can't stand the heat, then please excuse yourself from the table and Bee and I will continue our conversation," Dr. Moreland said with sarcasm and understatement.

"No, daddy, it's time for me to go to school," Bee retorted, as she got up and began to leave the table.

"Wait, Bee, we need to go, too," Jason added and all of the children left the room.

"Well Frank, the kids are seeing right through you. Do you have any idea how this is affecting them?" Jacqueline observed.

"Well, shit, I'm doing the best I can with what I've got. I'm going to Alcoholics Anonymous and trying to cut down on the drinking— looking for that day when I can put two days together without a drink," Frank said with conviction, hopefully avoiding what he knew would be another fight.

"OK, since I can't do it, maybe the kids will keep up the pressure for you to quit," she responded to Frank and, avoiding any further conversation, began to clear the breakfast table.

"I am going to quit when I am damn good and ready and no matter how much you say, no matter how biting you are, and no matter how much you try to turn the kids against me, I am going to live my life as I see fit, alcohol or no alcohol. And by the way, Blanch is not going anywhere either—and, you know, you can have a divorce any time you want it," he elaborated; but not for the first time did he explain himself and what he was going to do.

From the kitchen, Jacqueline added something she had said repeatedly, "Don't worry, when the kids are in college or away from the house, you can have your divorce —good riddance and thank God."

"Oh, yea, you can thank God, all right," he added as he got up from the table and turned to go out the door to start another day with the sick and infirm.

CHAPTER TWELVE

"...do you have a roommate?"

In the top of the fifteenth inning, Carolina broke through, scored a run, and won the game when Duke failed to score in the bottom of the inning. The visiting team received relatively quiet applause from a depleted crowd. The winning run began with a walk, putting a man on first base. He was the Carolina second baseman and was the fastest man on the team. Everyone in the stadium knew he was going to steal second base. With the count at two balls and a strike, he easily made it to second. Two outs later, the hero of the game, Jack Simmons, singled through the box and though the call at home plate was close, the man scored from second base. In the bottom half of the inning Carolina called on its best pitcher, after only three days rest, and he struck out the side. The game was over and Carolina was a leg-up on Duke. Those in light blue went home happy; one more win and their team would secure a second seed in the ACC tournament in Greensboro, North Carolina. Those in dark blue went home unhappy, but were thankful the series had two more games.

When the game was over, the Duke Frank, who had stayed through the whole game, came down to where Jackie was standing and started in, "I guess you know the business with the bottle really pissed me off!"

"Oh, yea, it was very obvious you were really pissed off," Jackie responded, looking straight at Frank and speaking with conviction, not meaning to back off, or in any way to seem passive. (Jackie was nearly as pissed off as Frank, particularly when he suffered the barrage of profanity Frank sent his way.)

"I think you owe me an apology—I wasn't hurting anybody and, for sure, I didn't have enough liquor to get drunk or be under the influence," Frank replied, an angry edge to his voice.

"Sorry, Frank, but I see no reason to apologize for responding to someone flagrantly breaking the rules and putting himself and others at risk. Rules are rules and maybe you didn't know you could not bring liquor into the ballpark and drink it," Jackie, in a calm demeanor, elaborated and added, "but that is no excuse, for I'm sure the same rule applies in your ballpark on the Duke campus."

Frank was turning red, about to lose his temper. He knew he had a quick trigger when he got mad. "Is it Jackie?" Frank asked, mature enough to know he had to temporize.

"Yes, you know my name is Jackie."

Frank hissed, "That's a girl's name."

"Don't push, Frank, none of this is worth losing your cool over and making sarcastic remarks," Jackie said, staying cool. They were nearly the only people left in the ballpark.

"OK, Jackie, we'll see what happens. Maybe we'll meet again," Frank said, turned and started down the steps to the exit ramp.

To Jackie, the last comment sounded like a threat. That comment raised several questions in his mind. How would he ever find me again—at a ballgame? Surely, there is no way he could find out where I live. Is there any way he could find out my academic schedule? Jackie hoped the answer to these questions was no, he couldn't possibly find out all these things.

One thing Jackie was sure of was that he wasn't going to the Bulls ballpark any time soon, and he surely wasn't ever going to the Duke ballpark.

Halfway through his graduate work in psychology, Jackie Moreland was called into service in the United States Navy. Through what was called the Berry Plan, he had been deferred from service until he was out of college. After a training course in grief management, he was assigned the position of Hospital chaplain at the Naval Hospital in Jacksonville, Florida. A First Lieutenant, he was certainly a greenhorn, but he learned quickly and became proficient in handling difficult cases that resulted from the loss of a close relative or friend. After college, Jackie had married a classmate who was his age and came from a family similar to his own. You may ask, "Was he in love?" Yes, of course, he was "in love."

But in Jacksonville it all began, barely a newlywed, he planned and experienced a long series of clandestine encounters with the opposite sex. There was no rhyme or reason to the liaisons, except the fact that the women were attractive and slim—which is to say he had no attraction to overweight, unattractive women. Of course, that says a lot about his long list of biases that plagued him his entire life. He lived two lives and his secret life was associated with profound guilt. He would right his "ship" each and every time only to fall into the trap of forbidden sex once again. He knew he had the "can't help its" and would vow each and every time that the last encounter was truly the last. Needless to say, he was in a vicious cycle.

Candace was in the American Red Cross, assigned to the same naval hospital as Jackie. On a Monday morning early in July, Candace was having coffee by herself in the hospital cafeteria. Clad in the pale blue of the ARC, she was pale-skinned with freckles. She was slim and had reddish-brown hair and small breasts. Was she unattached and lonely? No doubt Jackie was going to find out in hurry. He approached her table and said in a calm, low and confident voice, "May I sit with you?"

"Oh, please do," Candice said. She thought, *What an attractive Naval Officer! Dollars to donuts, he's married.* She quickly surveyed his left hand and saw the ring. Of course, that was a blessing and a curse, for she didn't have to worry about a serious commitment, but unfortunately the relationship was unlikely to last very long.

"I'm Jackie Moreland," he said, as he sat down across from her.

"Candace Morgan, "she responded.

"You're in the American Red Cross, right? What do you do here?" he asked and sipped a cup of black coffee.

"Right, I work in the admissions office helping patients get settled in their rooms."

"All right, sort of on the front line, I guess."

"Well, you might say so, but I feel like I'm a little undervalued," she responded, running her fingers around the edge of her coffee cup, a movement that was not lost on Jackie. Candace was single and had not had any relationship with a man in more than two years. She was thirty-three and lonely.

"No doubt, but maybe you'll be promoted into a more responsible position," Jackie said, keeping his hazel eyes pinned on his prey. He smiled, but not too much. He had been here before. He imagined her in her apartment, at the bar, her skirt hiked well above her knees.

"Lieutenant Moreland..."

"Please call me Jackie, Candace." It could have been his imagination, but it seemed to him that she was blushing and breathing faster. He kept his reactions to a minimum, hoping there would be time to let his emotions show.

"All right, Jackie, you're married, aren't you?" she asked, demurely looking down.

"Yes, I am. Does that turn you off or, maybe, it turns you on?" he asked, sensing a change in his groin.

"Well, I don't know. I certainly don't know you well enough, but you are an attractive man." God, she couldn't believe she said that. A little chill ran through her body and she could feel her nipples waking up. After a moment, she thought, *I can believe you said that—we're going so fast my head is spinning.*

"Thank you. You are an attractive woman. Do you live nearby?" With that question he was putting money on the table, hoping she lived by herself in an apartment deep in a subdivision.

"Ah...yes, I have an apartment behind the hospital," she hesitated, but her body was telling her that this meeting had real possibilities. His being married made her feel safer than if he had been single, but she knew she could be letting her emotions get away from her. She was going to ask him if he was a gentleman, who wouldn't take advantage of a vulnerable woman.

"What time do you get off work?" he asked, his confidence soaring.

"Today, I get off at four-thirty," she replied, a twinkle in her eye and an acquiescing tone in her voice.

"Candace, may I ask you a personal question?"

"Yes, of course, but I may not answer it." She wasn't sure why she answered the way she did, but she didn't want to come across as being easy, though she was.

"Are you in a serious relationship?"

"No, I'm not. I don't consider that too personal, since I know you are."

'How about this, do you have a roommate?"

"Yes, I do, but I think we can work around that," she said, positively. She was ready to come out of her dress.

"Look, I am on call tonight and have to stay in the hospital...could we get together later on this evening? I mean, do you have other plans?" Jackie didn't let on, but he should have asked about her plans before he asked about getting together.

"No, I don't have other plans and, yes, we can get together later this evening," she intoned with as much energy as she could gather. She might as well admit it, she was getting hot, very hot...she could feel it in her pants.

"Look, here's a good plan. It is very unlikely that I will get called after eight o'clock, so leave your uniform on and come by room 17 in the doctor's quarters any time after eight...how's that sound?"

"How do I ask this? Are you a gentleman and I mean, a g-e-n-t-l-e-m-a-n?"

"Yes, I am, but there is no question, you are taking a risk, as I am, but yours is greater, obviously," Jackie said with sincerity and confident eye contact.

"Well…your plan sounds good," Candace said with some hesitation.

"Look, at the very least we will get to know one another better, but let me be clear, I am not a demanding type who wouldn't take no for an answer, ok?"

"OK, we'll see you around eight."

"Honestly, you won't regret it and I can assure you, we'll come away as friends." Jackie got up and left the cafeteria, a definite bulge in his pants.

CHAPTER THIRTEEN

"She reached for the strings of his scrubs and pulled one of the ends."

After an early supper in the cafeteria and two calls with questions that he could answer over the phone, Jackie retired to his room with some paperwork and a risque novel. He came out of his uniform and got into some hospital scrubs. His room was small—he liked to considerate it intimate. On 'high alert' he couldn't help but think about Candace and what might transpire. Doubts always crept into these situations, but he was confident they would end up in bed. He checked the drawer in the night stand next to his bed for a condom he had stashed beneath his underwear. It was there. On purpose he set the thermostat up, raising the temperature to nearly seventy five degrees. He settled in with his novel and waited, nerves all jangled up.

Just after eight o'clock, there was a quiet knock on the door numbered seventeen. Jackie's jangled nerves spoke up and sent a river of electricity through his body. *Oh, good, good, good…"* he thought—*"it is going to happen!"* Opening the door, seeing Candace in her uniform, he said, "Hi!" in his sexiest voice.

She responded with an equally sexy voice, "Hi, yourself!"

He shut the door quietly and grabbed Candace and with great exhaling held her tight to his body. He was already juiced by the thrill that fueled his incredible desire. She responded positively, thrusting her pelvis into his and moving side to side, feeling a huge erection. Breaking the embrace, Candace turned around, giving Jackie a chance to unzip her uniform. He paused, then quickly realized that she wanted to come out of the dress and give him the view; she had no bra on. Making sure she felt his touch, he slowly unzipped her and moved his hands under the shoulders of her dress. She stepped out of the dress and turned to face him with only a pair of black panties on. She reached for the strings of his scrubs and pulled one of the ends. The bottoms did not fall—they were caught on an enormous erection. Jackie took a deep breath, tensed his abdominal muscles and the bottoms fell to the floor. Candace went down on Jackie and performed oral sex. After mutual organisms, Jackie took Candace to bed for old-fashioned sex. They slept through the night, awoke to the rising sun and had sex for a second time. Both showered and went their separate ways to work. As opposed to the prospect that this might be a one and done event, they continued to have sex on a regular basis in room seventeen.

CHAPTER FOURTEEN

"Oh, well, she must have suspected I would be available."

Statesville was not a country club town to speak of—it only had a tennis and swim club that was just getting started when Jackie moved there and set up his psychology practice. Since there was only one other psychologist with a degree in town, he anticipated a successful endeavor. Married with two children, Jackie had plenty of incentive to establish a thriving practice. And since he was a tennis player, he was a prime target for membership in the tennis and swim club; and that, along with joining a church, were important steps to getting him known in the community.

It had been one of those situations where one man owned a lot of land suitable for such a club. Money was no object when the idea for the club came to Alex Smitherman's attention. It didn't take much thought and analysis for Alex to make the club happen, but such actions had to be blessed by his attorney and investment advisor. He was also smart enough to know he had to stay in the background when it came to management of the club. Alex had sized up Jackie Moreland from the beginning and asked him to chair the club's board of directors: seven men and five women. Jackie jumped at the chance, particularly since the ground had already been broken for a small clubhouse, six composition (soft clay) tennis courts and an Olympic-sized swimming pool. With a known name and money be-hind the endeavor, Jackie knew this project was going to be successful.

The board of directors had an organizational meeting in March of the year the construction of the club began. They met in the library of a lawyer, Raymond Reynolds, who had a downtown office. All twelve members of the board were present. The first order of business was the election of officers of the board. Jackie Moreland was elected as President and Chair and Robin Smithwick as secretary. The elec-tion of officers was followed by the appointment of Jack Overland as chair of the membership committee, who was charged with filling in the six members that would begin the important job of recruiting new members to the club. Other committees included house and grounds, chaired by Raymond Reynolds, and a search committee for a tennis professional chaired by the President, who was also recognized as li-aison with Alex Smitherman.

From the other end of the table, Robin Smithwick caught the Chair's eye. She stared at him intently; her brown eyes straight ahead, her head never dropping. A slight smile was apparent too, and meant only for Jackie. This was not the look of a curious woman; this was the serious look of a woman intent on making contact with the object of her attention. It wasn't as if he hadn't seen this before, but consid-ering the circumstances related to the formation of the club, he per-ceived it as somewhat unusual. Also, it wasn't like he had not made social contact with Robin—they played tennis together every Sunday afternoon. He was hopeful that his instincts were correct: she was making a move to establish a relationship that would be physically and emotionally serious.

Robin fit the bill, she was outstandingly beautiful and physically trim. A brunette, she kept her hair short, neat and close to her head. Also, she dressed neatly and appropriately. Jackie would not call her full-bosomed—as a matter of fact she was flat-chested. That was of no matter to him, her breasts (or lack thereof) were offset by her beauty and intelligence. Jackie was sure of his instincts, but he had to confirm that with affirmation from the "horse's mouth." Since they moved in the same social circle, there would be no lack of contact, but that meant there would be only casual conversations—obviously they were going to have to meet secretly. Either way, this relationship was going to be fraught with tension, not only from the physical attraction itself, but also from the fact that it was going to be a liaison easily subjected to the risk of being detected.

At the end of the second board meeting as Robin had continued to make eye contact, she lingered around after everyone else had left, and she and Jackie struck up a conversation.

"You look fetching tonight, Robin," Jackie observed, his eyes locking in on hers.

She smiled, actually laughed, and responded, "Fetching? What do you mean by that?"

"Oh, you know what that means," he said, laughing at himself.

"Yes, I know what that means, but I think there are better words to use if you are giving a compliment," she said, knowing that if he thought she was beautiful, then he should say it in a more expressive way.

"OK, you are beautiful tonight, as always," he said the obvious, touching her arm.

"Now that's better and I thank you, and you don't look so bad yourself," she said, knowing that he was going to come back at her, objecting to the '...so bad yourself.'"

"Gag, I would have to repeat what you just said to me: there are better words with which to pay a compliment," he said, irony dripping on every word.

"OK, you are very handsome tonight, as always," she intoned, her dark brown eyes sparkling in the evening light.

"Thank you, yourself. May I make an observation? You have been staring at me ever since we began working together on the board," Jackie said.

"Was it that obvious?" she said demurely and then followed that with a chuckle.

"Yes, Ma'me, it was."

"Oh, God not the proverbial `Ma'me,' that is so southern."

"Well," he responded, "I'm sorry, please excuse me, but you know I am very southern."

"Jackie," she retorted, "I was staring because I find you interesting, as well as attractive,"Robin spoke with a forthrightness that most women would not use so early in a possibly budding relationship.

"Is it that obvious that I am so vulnerable?" Jackie said, blushing and looking down. He was beginning to consider the prospect for a serious relationship to be good, maybe excellent.

"I don't know about vulnerable, but I sensed that you might be—shall I say—available," she responded, knowing she had gone out on a limb and could be put in a very embarrassing situation.

"Wow, you don't mince around, do you? To put you at ease, yes, I am available—actually I would say 'very' available," he intoned with a broad smile and a chill to the bone. He wanted to grab her right then, but he simply took her hand in his. A tight squeeze was returned in kind.

"Tomorrow, at noon, in the Wiley School parking lot...we'll talk some more," she responded confidently, turned and went out he library door.

"Robin, wait," Jackie declared, "I need to check my calendar to see if I'm available."

Robin had already gone and probably didn't hear his declaration. He did like what he saw of her backside.

"She must have known I'd be available," Jackie commenting to himself, laughing simultaneously.

It was not lost on Jackie that Robin did not mention their weekly tennis game. He surmised she wanted to keep their new and budding romance distinct and separate from the tennis, which was entirely social and involved both their families.

CHAPTER FIFTEEN

"Robin, you've been watching too much CSI."

To Jackie, there are two categories of chasing skirts: one he calls the minor leagues and the one he calls the major leagues. It all depends on what is known as social stratification: lower and higher levels of social interaction. A liaison with his secretary, he would consider a lower level; and an affair with Robin, he would consider a higher level. He is not being a social snob, but it all depended on the risk each party was taking. Phyllis, his secretary, is recently divorced with children; Robin is married with children. They both are risky endeavors—one or the other player is taking a chance on getting caught and exposed. But the consequences are greater at the major league level, particularly if the husband or the wife finds out. Robin and Jackie's wife are in the same social strata and that just makes the risks even greater. Take any scenario and you can see what the risks and consequences would be. One of the major differences is the fact that a relationship outside of marriage can become serious and pressure builds to dissolve one or both of the marriages. So it becomes pretty sticky if only one of the participants gets serious and wants out of his or her marriage. Here to fore, Jackie had avoided getting involved with anyone who was in his social strata. If he thought about it at all, he would avoid an affair with an attractive woman he socialized with, but when he is thinking with the organs below his waist, chances are, he'd take the risk.

Jackie took his lunch break from twelve to one o'clock. He left his practice a few minutes early and drove to Wiley School. He knew that Robin drove a distinctly dark-colored SUV and he saw the vehicle when he turned into the parking lot. A lump came into this throat; he realized then what a chance he was taking. He took a deep breath and parked beside Robin, who was surveying the school in front of her. He hadn't really thought about it, but he knew it would be up to him to get into her car.

He scanned the playground, looking for adults and saw only children; he scanned the parking lot and saw only empty cars, concluding it was safe to get into Robin's car.

"Well, I wasn't sure you would come, but here you are and you're all dressed up," Robin opened the conversation in a relatively low, but positive, voice.

Jackie took in the sight and aroma of a fantastically beautiful woman and responded, "I decided I really couldn't think about it—all I knew was I wanted to see you again. And, you look very nice yourself and you smell good, too." She took his breath away.

What in the world did this uncommonly good-looking woman want with me? It makes me wonder how things were with her at home, he thought. *Caroline, my wife, and I were thrown with Robin and Bill at every social event, including the aforementioned Sunday afternoon tennis. Statesville was not a big town and there were really only one consistent social group and we were in it.*

"Is this your regular lunch hour?" Robin asked, thinking, you know, this is one very attractive man and I'm falling all over myself to be in his arms.

"Yes, it is. I have patients from nine until eleven in the morning, leaving me time to go over my notes before lunch. I start again at two and finish with patients by four o'clock. I'm usually home by five-thirty."

"What do you think about me being one of your patients?" she asked, turning toward Jackie, her dress above her knees.

He was shocked and caught his breath, answering with a few moments hesitation, "I'd have to think about that. Are you serious?"

"I'm very serious, but I realize that psychologists don't have affairs with their patients," she retorted, her voice, simply, extremely appealing.

"So, right off the bat, before I've really thought about it, do you want to be my patient or do you want to have an affair," he asked, very aware of her body language.

"Both, but if I had to choose one or the other, I would take an affair," she said, holding his hand and looking longingly into his eyes. Then, before he could respond, she added, "I don't see why I couldn't be your patient in your office and your concubine in a motel room."

"You don't mean 'concubine' do you? How about just being lovers?" Jackie asked, as he took her hand and kissed it. He didn't know about Robin, but he felt the sexual tension in the air—it gave him chills and goose bumps. He wanted her badly and he sensed she felt the same way.

"I'd like that, but where are we going to do it so that we can feel safe?" she asked, concern in her voice.

"I think I can solve that problem. My secretary and receptionist, Phyllis, lives on a farm with an out building set up as an office. She has recently been divorced and the office is not being used. We can rendezvous there."

"Well, how do you know it would be available?" she asked with a knowing smile and a squeeze of his hand.

"Oh, I don't, but I think I know her well enough to ask if it would be available. The only problem is we would have to do it when her kids are in school and I don't know their schedule," he responded, returning the squeeze.

"OK, write down my cell phone number—no, memorize it and call me from a pay phone," she instructed him.

"You've been watching too much CSI, Robin, but it's not a bad idea. Let's do the same with my cell," he said back.

CHAPTER SIXTEEN

"Are you nuts? I'll meet you tomorrow."

Jackie's secretary, Phyllis Turner, was a divorcee with two children in grammar school. Slim and attractive, she came to work neatly trimmed and boasting short blonde hair. For a short time immediately after he began his practice, he and Phyllis were lovers, but over the months the sexual tension diminished and she began seeing another man. Actually that was all right with Jackie, since the relationship was awkward and there would be no future to it. By that time, they had started what would eventually be a deep friendship based on respect and love, but not sex. Each leaned on the other for emotional support. An open relationship, they kept no secrets. Phyllis knew about Robin from the beginning and warned Jackie about the risks he was taking if he and Robin started a "full-blown" affair.

It was a warm, sunny Monday when Jackie broke the news to Phyllis that, yes, indeed, he and Robin had decided they wanted to engage in a deeply personal and intimate relationship. Unfortunately, they had no place in which to consummate the affair.

"Phyllis, Robin and I need your help. Is it possible for us to use your outside office for our meetings? It would have to be at lunch time and when we were sure your kids were in school or otherwise occupied," Jackie explained, opening their conversation first thing that morning when there were no patients in the waiting room.

"You're really going to do it, huh?" Phyllis asked.

"Yep, we are," Jackie answered quickly with no hesitation.

"Sure, you can use the office building," she answered, raising her eyebrows to let him know she still had reservations about the affair, considering it a great risk. "I'll have to be aware of your schedule, so I can be sure the kids will not be around. I know now that the kids will be in school the lunch hours for the rest of this week.

"Oh, don't worry, you'll be aware of our schedule and, furthermore, I want you to meet Robin. You'll like her. So, I haven't confirmed this with Robin, but we'll surely meet in the next day or two," Jackie responded with enthusiasm.

Robin was in the grocery store with her two kids the next day afternoon when her cell phone went off.

"Hello," she answered right away.

"It is I in a pay phone. Can you talk?"

"No, I can't, but call me back in an hour," she responded in a near whisper.

"No problem. I'll talk to you between patients around three o'clock," Jackie replied, emotionally prepared for any kind of unexpected interruption or delay in their plans.

Robin, with a sixth sense, could tell he had good news and that excited her—she immediately started thinking about what she was going to wear, knowing she could not wear perfume or makeup.

She thought to herself, *The dress will have to be loose, bright, and well above the knees.*

Her cell phone rang again at three o'clock and she answered, "Hello."

"It is all set up. Do you want to meet tomorrow or Wednesday?" he replied and, as a gentleman, gave her a choice.

"Are you nuts? I'll meet you tomorrow," she said with excitement in her voice. She added, "Just tell me what time and how to get there."

He responded without a pause, "Twelve noon...to get there, go west on Interstate Forty and about two miles out you will come to, believe it or not, Old Statesville Road. Bear right onto Old Statesville, and at about two more miles look for mailbox 1308 on your right. It's a gravel driveway which splits in two: the left fork takes you to Phyllis' home, and the right fork takes you to the office. You'll know you are at the office by the dark siding and black roof. Since the little office sits in a stand of pines, you can pull around to the back and you will be out of sight. You know the rules, don't you?"

"Yes, I know the rules—just don't expect me to be ready for an evening out on the town," she giggled.

Tuesday, a spring day in Piedmont, North Carolina, was warm and sunny at twelve noon. Excited and a little early, Robin got to the out building before Jackie and parked, as he suggested, in the back. The door to the "office" was unlocked and she went into the one-room building, which had a desk, a highback chair, and a daybed. The floor was covered, wall to wall, by a champaign-colored carpet. To one side there was a small sink with hot and cold-running water, but there were no bathroom facilities. Robin noted the latter and told herself she couldn't drink before she came, and, if there was wine available, she would have to be careful how much and how fast she drank.

Within five minutes, a soft knock was heard at the door. Robin was not prepared for the moment—she didn't know whether to respond vocally or to go and open the door. She didn't have to make a decision, as Jackie opened the door and stepped into the room.

"Hi, there!" he exclaimed, reaching for her.

They hungrily embraced, hard and tight. It was like, after years of separation, they had finally found each other.

"Hi, yourself," she replied, blowing out the air she had held until they parted. Breathlessly, she added, "There is no bathroom and that may not be a problem for you, but I am not going in the woods if the need arises.

"Well, you know, baby, I almost brought us a bottle of wine, but Phyllis reminded me that the carpet was of a light color and so I decided against it—we should bless this meeting with a kiss."

Robin came to him with uplifted face and he immediately saw she had no makeup on and was relieved, telling himself he wasn't going to mention it. Their lips met and each explored the other's mouth—neither was disappointed, and each felt the pelvic pressure they had generated. There was so much generated heat and they were so tightly meshed, they couldn't break away. Jackie took advantage of their closeness and went under her dress, slipped his hand under her panties, and took them down. For her part, she was nearly crazed with desire and she helped him take her panties down the rest of the way. Robin was the first to break away, and she immediately slipped out her dress in one smooth motion. She then undid his belt, unzipped his pants and, in one quick movement, took his pants down. They could hardly get their breath, but they knew they had to get to the daybed and make hard, passionate love, thrusting with a force that matched their desire for each other. Each reached a climax so quickly that both of them were slightly disappointed, but that would only mean the next time would be even more fantastic. The sexual tension was immediately released, and they held each other like there would be no next time.

It was time to go and it was also time, unfortunately, for Jackie to be beset with a soul-crushing guilt. But it wasn't like he didn't expect it, for he had been in this situation so many times before. Yet, even he sensed something different that would blunt the guilt. And, clearly, this was a defining relationship—both participants with children— that was seriously way beyond what either had experienced before.

"I'll call you tomorrow—for a first rendezvous, this was an incredible experience," Jackie said, kissing her lightly on the lips, his hands on both of her shoulders.

Both dressed and made their way out of the "office." They smelled like sex—both were going to have to shower before making any other human contact. But it was little bother, sinse sex had been so intense and, for them, out-of-this-world. Neither could wait for the next clandestine meeting.

CHAPTER SEVENTEEN

"...Sunday morning coming down."

The next Sunday morning in Statesville was very quiet and still—an unusual June day with a clear, cool beginning. Jackie, Caroline, and the two children visited the First Presbyterian Church for the eleven o'clock service. The sermon was on the feeding of the five thousand: the Reverend Beverly Jackson, a man, expounded on the miracle and it was his interpretation that, including the women and children, the crowd was actually closer to thirteen thousand. He elected not to give the miracle a rational explanation—it was simply inexplicable, except to say it was a miracle that came from God through Jesus.

After the church service and a quick lunch, the entire Moreland family changed into their tennis attires and went over to the Smithwick's for the adults to play mixed doubles and the children to play badminton. Even though Bill and Robin had built their house in a cul-de-sac, they had purchased two lots and placed the house in the middle of the now larger lot. That left considerable room for the tennis court, which was fenced in and featured a rubberized hard surface. The direction of the court was parallel to the house, and in between the court and the house was an outdoor round table with four matching chairs. Robin had set out a pitcher of lemonade and six glasses.

Jackie parked the car in front of the house, and he and his family came around to the back where Robin and Bill were warming up on the tennis court. The children, ranging in age from seven to nine years, settled in and played their badminton.

"Of course, you know that's not fair: warming up before the guests arrive," Jackie chided Robin and Bill.

"Well, hello to you, too, and welcome to our home," Bill responded, almost yelling.

Robin kept her eyes on the tennis ball; Jackie marveled at her consistent forehand. She had on a lavender tennis dress—low cut with a short skirt—captivating would be putting it mildly. Even though she seemed to concentrate on hitting the ball, Jackie caught her eyes between shots. Yes, it was weird and awkward, but somehow they managed to play along with what was a social event. Robin left the court and went over to welcome Caroline, who was in a very attractive dress of her own.

"Hi, Caroline, glad you, Jackie, and the kids could come over. Your dress is so cute—if your tennis is as good as you outfit, we don't stand a chance."

"Hey, Robin, you've seen my game; it's not nearly as good as yours," Caroline said, as she gave Robin a brief hug.

"Oh, Caroline, I'm already sweating," Robin said as she backed away from her guest and added, "How about some lemonade?"

"That would be great," Caroline said, as she and Robin went over to the table where the lemonade and glasses were. "Gosh," Caroline gushed, "I love your outfit—very stylish and attractive. You are such a handsome woman."

"Now, coming for you, that is a compliment of the first order, thank you," Robin responded.

Naturally competitive, the foursome became engaged in a spirited first set. Jackie was better than Bill and Robin was better than Caroline, so it was a close match. With the score tied at three games apiece, Bill stopped playing and stared out at the street in front of the house where there was a long black car, a Cadillac Escalade, the extended model. Two shadowy figures, presumably men, occupied the front seat. What Bill, or anybody else for that matter, did not know was that the car was well away from the curb with the motor running.

Bill spoke up, "Folks, believe it or not, there is a big black car in front of the house—to tell you the truth, I though you only saw these beasts on TV crime shows, or of course, in shady sections of New York, Chicago or Los Angeles. But I'm told you cannot be sure whether or not they are police detectives in casual clothes or thugs dressed to kill. I think I'll go over and say, "Howdy."

Robin immediately interjected, "Bill, I can't let you do that!"

"Honey, I assure you, they will move on if I look like I'm going over there, my racquet in my hand."

Sure enough, the two presumed men drove off when Bill started over there. "See, I told you they would skedaddle if someone started over there," Bill concluded.

Jackie questioned, "What in the world would they be doing in a quiet subdivision in Statesville? You know, I don't believe our cops drive that car—actually I know they don't."

"I don't know about the rest of you guys, but I think—no, I know—they are not from around here," Caroline observed.

"I agree with that," Bill said, "they are not from around here and, TV or not, I don't believe they were up to anything good."

"Has anybody done anything—like getting into an argument with a stranger—that might draw this kind of attention, this kind of response?" Bill asked.

"Well, it was years ago when I got into a confrontation with a Duke fan at a baseball game," Jackie admitted and added, "Now that doesn't sound like something that would bring out the bad guys, but I have to admit the Duke fan was mad as hell and he even threatened to 'see me again.'"

"I agree," Bill added and asked, "that doesn't sound like a threat that someone would hold onto and follow up with years later—were you in college"

"Yes, I was an undergraduate student at the University of North Carolina. How it all started was the fact that this Duke fan had brought a small bottle of whiskey into the game, and he took it out and had a swig. I made one of his friends get the bottle and throw it away in the men's room. The Dukie's name was Frank, and he cursed me with the f-word and the a-word the rest of the game. We went face to face after the game, and that's when he threatened me," Jackie summated.

Robin joined in the conversation, "I don't suppose anybody else has had such a run-in with somebody who would hire some thugs to come out here and intimidate us—if that is all they intended to do."

"I haven't, that's for sure," Caroline added.

"OK, let's do our due diligence. It probably doesn't mean anything, but let's keep a watch out for any unusual activity like strange cars parked in front of the house, particularly those that are long and black. But unfortunately, I would bet there is more than one car, or I wouldn't put it past them to put a new coat of paint on this car and the same goes for the license plate," Bill summed up.

"Bill, let's you and I discuss this with some neutral person, particularly someone who deals with these things a lot," Jackie added.

Bill responded, "I know just the right person, and he may want to hear your story again and get a description of the Duke fan who threatened you," and added, "I'll call you after I talk to my man." Bill broke away from the group and headed toward the house.

CHAPTER EIGHTEEN

"...a rather mild misunderstanding..."

The next day, Monday, came in like a house afire: heavy wind and rain sweeping savagely against a black sky. Bill Smithwick's power went out, along with the phones, but he had a cell phone on which he spent most of the morning. Jack Christian, a local freelance operative and detective, returned his call.

"Hello," Bill answered the call, anticipating who it might be.

"Bill, this is Jack Christian."

Bill responded, "Jack, thanks for returning my call. We have an unusual circumstance that may require your expertize."

"OK, go ahead, shoot," Jack came back to him.

"One of my friends, Jackie Moreland, who lives here in Statesville, has potentially serious problem," Bill started in and then added, "Two figures, presumably men, in a long black late-model Cadillac SUV, appeared and paused in front of my house. It occurred when we were playing tennis, and based on an old incident, it appears they were following Jackie. Now, the incident, on the surface, appears to be just a rather mild misunderstanding at a baseball game between Duke and North Carolina. Jackie had a Duke fan named Frank give up his whiskey bottle to one of his associates, who discarded the bottle in the men's room. The associate's name was Larry Bumgardner; he could confirm the incident and conversation that went on between Frank and Jackie."

"OK, go on."

"Larry, Frank, and two other guys, who were Carolina fans, had come to the game from work. So it was obvious to Jackie that they were out of college. Jackie, himself, was an undergraduate student at North Carolina at the time. Larry, upon the word of Jackie, made Frank give up the bottle and Larry discarded it in the men's room. Frank was outraged and kept up a string of profanities toward Jackie that included the f-word and the a-word. Jackie was uncomfortable, but he stayed at the game, which went into the fifteenth inning!"

"You know, there was a big write-up in the paper about the game...I believe it was in Durham at the Bulls' park," Jake observed and then asked, "Were the two men shabbily or reasonably well-attired?"

"I don't know, but I got the impression they were well-attired, but casual. Apparently, Frank and one other guy had on dark blue baseball caps marked with a big 'D.'"

"Was there a more serious altercation?" Jake asked.

"Yes, at the end of the game Frank came down to where Jackie was standing, got in his face, cursed him, and apparently said something like, `I'll see you again,' or 'You have not heard the last of this,'" Bill explained.

"I agree, it sounds fairly innocuous to me, but we need to find out whom the guys in the black car were following, assuming they were following somebody. Have Jackie reach me at this cell phone number and I'll take it from here. You know both good and bad guys travel in long black cars and, usually, in pairs," Jake elaborated.

"You're right about that if the TV shows are in the least bit realistic," Bill said, ready to hang up, but he added, "I'll have Jackie call you."

In the meantime, the two male persons in the long black car parked in a downtown parking lot and went over the events of that Sunday. The driver, a man named Blake, looked over at his partner, a man named Whitey. They were both Caucasian and dressed casually in slacks and short-sleeved shirts. Their age was somewhere between thirty and forty. Both wore a neatly trimmed mustache and goatee, set on prematurely wrinkled sunbaked skin. The car carried the tell-tale scent of cigarette smoke—they were chain-smokers, lighting up like they were paired twins. Each had a nine-millimeter Glock under the car seat and knew how to handle and shoot it—every six months they went to the firing range to hit at least nine out of ten bull's eyes.

"Well, that was real exciting," Blake said sarcastically in reference to their outing in front of Bill Smithwick's house.

"Yea, real exciting, and what did that damn fool think he was going to do? It reminded me of the old dog who chased cars and never caught them," Whitey said and then added, "It made me smile to think how he would have shit in his pants, if we did no more than shoot up in the air."

"Oh yea, that would have been funny, but you know we haven't been given clear instructions as to what we are supposed to do, if one of them were to come too close to the car," Blake observed.

"It was my understanding that we were supposed to scare them—say nothing, look mean and menacing, maybe show a gun, but nothing more. If we did say something, it was not to let them know we were after one of the men," Whitey explained, sitting in the so-called 'shot-gun seat.'

"You know what I think—I think there are too many cooks in the kitchen. What has filtered down to us has been so diluted out that we don't know what our responsibilities are. It was never clear to me as to whether or not we were supposed to scare them with gunfire. And since it is against the law to discharge a weapon inside the city limits, we could have been arrested. I wonder what it was that this Jackie Moreland has done. Supposedly it was some years ago and this Frank somebody has carried a grudge all these years. What the hell has he been doing all this time?" Blake carried on.

"Well, you missed it. It took this Frank that long to find out who it was that pissed him off. It had something to do with a drink of whiskey," Whitey said, trying to clarify the situation.

"OK, let's part company. I'll put this baby away so that nobody can find it—that fool that chased us might have gotten our license plate, so I'll have to change tags. Incidentally, are we to assume that the one who acted like he was going to accost us was this Morehead fellow?" Blake asked.

"I made that assumption, but I could be dead wrong. I do know he would be able to identify this car—as if this Escalade in this town wouldn't draw a lot of attention. We need some instructions as to whether or not we should change cars," Whitey observed and then added, "I don't think changing the color of the car will help us at all."

Jackie dialed Jack Christian's cell phone number and got a quick response, "This is Jack Christian."

"Jack, this is Jackie Moreland. I'm a friend of Bill Smithwick. He told me you could probably help me with a sticky problem."

"Well, as you can imagine, in some cases I can be very helpful, but in other cases I am no help at all," Jack responded honestly, as he was blowing smoke from a cigarette.

"That's fair enough. I and my family were at Bill Smithwick's playing tennis when two figures, presumably men, in a long black car drove slowly by, maybe even stopped, but they were well away from the curb. The windows were tinted so that you could not see the figure's faces, but Bill saw enough to conclude they were not wearing caps.

"Bill was able to get the license plate number, which was a North Carolina tag numbered SBG¬1066. The only thing that I could add was that the car had mag wheels with broad tires. Oh, yes, it was clean, easily reflecting the bright sun that fell on that Sunday. Bill said the car was a very late-model Cadillac Escalade, the extended variety."

"OK, how did you know they were looking for you? That is, assuming they were looking for somebody in particular."

"Well, actually I don't know for certain they were looking for me, but, of the four adults there, I was the only one who could remember having a confrontation with a stranger,"

"Now, tell me about this confrontation with a stranger," Jack requested, seeking as much information as possible.

Jackie paused, thought a second or two, and then said, "It occurred at a Duke/North Carolina baseball game. Sometime, right after the game started, four relatively young men came down the steps to my section right behind first base. Three of them sat a few rows behind me. The fourth sat next to me and I introduced myself to him, 'Hi, I'm Jackie Moreland."

He replied, "Hi, I'm Larry Bumgardner."

I said, "I'm glad to meet you, are you a Duke fan? I asked.

"Well, yes and no. I went to school back east at Dartmouth, but I have sort of adopted the Blue Devils."

"What about the other guys?" I asked.

"Two of them are graduates of North Carolina, the other is a Duke graduate," Larry explained. "OK, tell me what happened, or as they say, 'what transpired."

Jack briefly interrupted him. Jackie sighed and told the story once again, "The Duke graduate named Frank had brought a small bottle of an alcoholic beverage to the game and soon after it started he brought the bottle out and had a swig or two. I told Larry what Frank had brought with him and that he had taken one or more swigs from the small bottle. I also told Larry that Frank could be thrown out of the ballpark, if one of the security people found out what he had brought to the game and that he was drinking from it. Larry went up to Frank and took the bottle away from him and went and discarded it in the men's room."

"So far, so good. Surely that's not the end of the story," Jake surmised.

"No, it was not the end of the story. Apparently, Larry told Frank that I had seen him drink from the bottle and had presumed it contained an alcoholic beverage other than beer. Well, that pissed Frank off to no end and he cursed me using the f-word and the a-word the whole game," Jackie continued the story.

"That doesn't sound like much of a confrontation to me," Jake noted.

"No, it doesn't, not at that juncture. The so-called 'confrontation' occurred after the game was over, all fifteen innings of it. Frank came down to where I had stood up to go and got in my face with more of the same profanity. In no uncertain terms, he made it clear that I had really pissed him off and he was not going to be satisfied until I apologized. I said I wasn't about to apologize for saving his neck and keeping him in the ballpark," Jackie explained in a monotone.

Then Frank said, "Well, if that is the case, then you have not seen or heard the last of me," he said with conviction and a threatening tone of voice. He then turned and joined the rest of his party who had been waiting, just in case there was going to be fisticuffs.

"So how long has it been since this face-to-face confrontation took place?" Jake questioned Jackie.

"It was in April, two years ago," Jackie answered.

"So, no phone calls, no letters, no summons or any other means of contact since then?"

"Nothing, no contact of any kind. Had there been any kind of surveillance? Not that I or my family know of."

"OK, then, let me take it from here. I don't have to tell you to call me should you be contacted in any way or if you see another long black late-model car slow down in front of your or Bill's house. Tell me that license plate number again," Jake was finishing up, at least for this segment of the investigation.

"North Carolina license plate number SBG-1066," Jackie said, realizing that the next time he was to see that car, it would have another license plate and, maybe, another color.

It was late on the Monday after the incident that occurred in front of Bill Smithwick's house.

Blake, one of the shadowy figures in the long black car, responded to the ring of his cell phone, "Hello."

"Blake, where are you and can you talk?" a deep voice asked.

"I'm at my father's farm and, yes, I can talk," Blake answered.

"Where is the Escalade?" the deep voice asked a second time.

"In my father's barn," Blake answered, this time with an unsteady voice.

"And the license plate?"

"Battered and buried deep in the adjacent woods," Blake said, his voice continuing to break down.

"OK, good. Now you know not to try to contact me in any way or at all costs," the voice said, still deep and resonant.

"Right, I won't—actually I can't—try to contact you. But you should know it is not exactly clear what we are to do, if anything," Blake pointed out, his voice somewhat back together.

"I understand that, but you should know that I know about as much as you do about this surveillance. Obviously, we are trying to scare Jackie Moreland and his friends. Under no circumstance should you fire your weapon, and don't let them get close enough to be able to give the police a description of you and Whitey. Now, do you have the wherewithall to change the color of the car?"

"Yes, right here on the farm, right here in the barn," Blake responded.

"What color paint are you going to use?"

"Burgundy," Blake answered with a more optimistic voice.

"And you have another license plate to use?" the voice asked in an even deeper tone. "Yes."

"What is the number? I assume it is a North Carolina tag."

"JKA-2022, but it is a South Carolina tag.

"All right, here is your assignment: place Jackie Moreland's office under surveillance, but do not show your face. Furthermore, we have been ordered to photograph every person that goes in or out of that office. Those who are giving the orders are particularly interested in any woman going in or out of that office."

"Any woman in particular?" Blake inquired.

"Like I said, any woman going in or out of the office. It is best you not know who is going in or out of that office."

"So, we are not going to follow Jackie Moreland anymore?" Blake asked, curiosity getting the best of him.

"If our informants are correct, there is a connection between a certain woman and this Jackie Moreland."

"So you mean this Moreland guy is having an affair with a woman who is one of his patients?" Blake asked, now his curiosity getting the best of him.

"Look, smart guy, just do as you are told—and I might add, paid handsomely—and photograph all persons who go in and out of that office."

"I thought you said just women."

"I got a text that said to monitor and photograph all persons who go in or out of that office. At the distance you'll be working from, you may not be able to tell whether the 'patient' is a man or a woman, particularly a man in drag. Now, you two are to get on the job and don't forget your telescopic lens."

In the meantime, the "major league affair" continued to progress and took on a life of its own. Jackie and Robin were stuck in the web of deceit, but the lust they had for each other blinded them to the reality of an extra-marital affair that could only end badly. Bill Smithwick was beginning to suspect Robin, his wife, of infidelity, but he waited for concrete evidence. He hired a private investigator who staked out her car and followed her to the "office," where he was able to identify Jackie Moreland's car. In less than two weeks, his job was done—that's the long and short of it. What was Bill going to do about his wife's infidelity?

Actually, Bill wasn't surprised Robin was having an affair, but he was shocked when he learned that her partner in deceit was Jackie Moreland. The hurt poisoned Bill's mind—his thoughts ranged from self-administered death to murder. He quickly rejected any thoughts of suicide for that would give Robin, he thought, too much pleasure and license to carry on with the affair, even maybe to marry a man who he thought was a friend. But, first, before he decided what he was going to do, he accosted Robin one evening after supper when the kids had gone to bed.

"Robin, we need to talk," Bill started up, a neutral tone in his voice. The gravity of the situation was not lost on him, however.

"I'm tired, Billy, what is it you want to talk about?" Robin didn't like how he started the conversation, which is to say he never started one with "we have to talk." She was immediately suspicious and defensive, suspecting he may have discovered that she was seeing somebody on the sly. However, she was determined to deny it until he came up with enough sorted details to convince her he knew who it was that she was seeing.

"Oh, I don't think this will take too long, since I know who you are having an affair with," Bill responded, doing his best to remain calm.

"What? Me, having an affair? You can't be serious," she said, her back up, knowing she could intimidate him, even with body language.

"I'm as serious as a heart attack," he remarked back to her with a conviction she had not witnessed before. His tone was one of "you're not going to intimidate me any longer."

"OK, smarty-pants, with whom am I having an affair?"

"Jackie Moreland," he answered with confidence.

"Oh, come on, you don't really think I am seeing Jackie, one of our best friends," she said with a firm tone that would usually make Bill back off—it wasn't the first time he had suspected her of seeing somebody else.

"I've got the goods on you this time. I had a private detective follow you to the meeting place, an outhouse in the country that belongs to Jackie's secretary," Bill elaborated, beginning to feel anger he was determined not to show.

"You had a private detective follow me? Why? What in the world convinced you to do that?" Robin asked, for the first time showing deviance.

"Well, it was mostly my intuition, because there were days when you didn't wear any makeup," Bill said, with an ever increasing confidence. He knew eventually she would have to admit to having the affair.

"You know that doesn't mean anything—often I go without makeup," she said, realizing she was losing the battle.

"Robin, how long are you going to deny this, when I have incontrovertible evidence that you are seeing Jackie?" he questioned, trying to cover up his losing of patience.

"All right, damn it, I'm seeing Jackie. What are you going to do about it?" Robin asked, irritation in her voice.

"Well, you don't have to get snotty showing deviance in your voice. I have already talked to a lawyer about your behavior, because I'm not going to accept this lying down. I'm filing for a divorce, and in the meantime you have to move out of the house," Bill said with authority in his tone of voice.

"I'll be damned. I'll get my own lawyer and you can have your divorce. But I'm not leaving this house."

"We'll see about that, because, according to my lawyer, you don't have any choice in the matter," Bill responded, feeling the tension rising in the air.

"Yes, we'll see about that, especially since I own half of the house," Robin said, again with deviance in her voice.

"Well, that's about what I expected from you. I have a feeling this is going to take some time to settle. In the meantime, you can have the spare bedroom, and it will be your responsibility to tell the children why you are sleeping in the spare bedroom," Bill said, finality in his voice.

CHAPTER NINETEEN

"...surveillance abruptly cancelled..."

Blake and Whitey were on the job, watching Jackie Moreland's office. Their instructions were to be inconspicuous and photograph all persons going in and out of the office, but there was little activity and few persons to photograph.

"God, this is boring," Blake observed, breaking the silence.

"You know, I think I can recognize the four tennis players we saw last Sunday, and except for Jackie Moreland, none of them has gone into his office," Whitey replied.

Blake's cell phone rang and he answered, "Hello."

"Blake, the surveillance has been called off. Get out of there now and lie low," the deep voice rang out with authority.

"Yes, sir," Blake answered, "We are out of here."

Blake and Whitey drove away from the office; there was no chance they were or could have been seen. Once again, Blake parked the car in his father's barn. He and Whitey followed instructions and laid low.

The incessant rain stopped and a bright sun came out, raising the spirits of the people of Statesville and the surrounding environs. Jackie had finished two sessions with patients the second Wednesday after the tennis game was interrupted by the presence of a surveillance car. He was working over his notes when his cell phone went off.

"Hello, this is Dr. Moreland," he said, his tone and voice volume reduced in case it was a personal call, i.e., Robin.

"Jackie, Robin."

"Yes, baby, I hoped you would call—as a matter of fact, I was going to call you after my morning sessions."

"Well, you'd be wasting your breath, because you and I are history," Robin announced, about to break up, emotionally.

"We are history? What does that mean? We have just gotten started," Jackie responded with a slight edge to his voice, refusing to believe what was happening.

"Bill had me followed, and the detective was able to identify both of our cars and observed us when we both came out of the office," Robin explained, reluctantly.

"Jesus, Robin, how did Bill take it—actually I can imagine what he said and how he must have felt," Jackie responded.

"Yes, about as well as you could have expected—he was sad, mad, and mystified. He probably didn't recognize it, but he balled up his fists. The first verbal reaction was he was going to throw me out of the house, but, since I own half of the house, he had no right to do that. I was, however, banished to the spare bedroom, which at the time I had no way to object to it since it seemed perfectly logical we certainly couldn't sleep together—neither of us wanted to do that considering the fact I had just torn up the marriage. I'm not going to stay very long in the house, if he makes my life miserable.

"Robin, Bill can't stop us from seeing each other, can he?" Jackie asked, a desperate tone to his voice.

"No, but my lawyer can—and he has," Robin responded in resignation.

"Well, I'm sorry. I had hoped we could carry on for some time. Even though it will be from a distance, I will always love you. Maybe someday we will be able to see each other. 1 hope and pray that Caroline won't find out about this, but no bigger than Statesville, the prospect of keeping it under wraps is rather dim. Honey, thanks for the call, and remember I will think of you constantly," Jackie elaborated.

"It has occurred to me, Jackie, that you might as well be the one to tell Caroline—you know, it is sometimes best if bad news comes from the horse's mouth."

Jackson, Jackson, and Jackson was a family law firm in Winston-Salem, North Carolina. It was touted to be one of the best firms in the state known for handling divorce cases. Bill Smithwick had gone to school with the youngest Jackson, and he was the first person Bill called when Robin admitted she was having an affair with Jackie Moreland.

"Jackson, Jackson, and Jackson, attorneys-at-law, how may I direct your call?" Mary, the receptionist, asked when she received the call.

"My name is Bill Smithwick. May I speak to Lawrence Jackson the Third?"

"Yes, you may. Please hold while I buzz his office," Mary said in a definitive voice.

"Hello, this Lawrence the Third. May I help you?"

"Larry, this is Bill Smithwick. I have some bad news: Robin has admitted to an affair. I wanted to throw he out of the house, but since the house is in both of our names, I don't think I can pull that off, can I?"

"You could do that only if there was a prior agreement that stipulated that in the event of infidelity, the house automatically goes to the harmed spouse. So far no such document exists—am I correct?" Larry answered.

"You are correct, there is no such document. For what it's worth, she has agreed to sleep in the spare bedroom until the divorce is settled or until she decides to move out on her own. It is a very tense situation and when she told the kids, the tension just got that much worse. They asked why she was going to move into the spare bedroom, but Robin only said that since she didn't love their father anymore, there was going to be a divorce. I don't think this misrepresentation of the facts is likely to stand up. I must admit I am contemplating telling the kids the whole story myself." Bill sighed as his voice tailed off.

"I agree her explanation won't likely stand up, but let some time go by before you spill the truth to the kids," Larry advised.

After a few silent moments had gone by, Bill asked, "When do you want to see me? What materials do I need to get together?"

Larry responded to Bill's question, "I tell you what. I think we will probably have some time before there is a meeting of both of you and us lawyers. Normally, I would ask for all your legal documents, but, since they were drawn up here in this office, I'll pull the appropriate documents and have them ready for your and mine's first meeting," Larry stated.

Bill's meeting with his lawyer occurred the second Wednesday after Robin admitted to the affair. It seemed like everything was wet from the rains, and the dense clouds keep the sunlight away.

"Bill, I have to ask you two questions before we do anything else. One, are you having, or have you ever had, an affair?" Larry asked.

"No, absolutely not on both counts," Bill replied without hesitation and with conviction.

"Two, have you ever physically accosted Robin or have you ever been on a campaign to emotionally berate her for little things that come up in a marriage?"

"No, definitely not, on both counts," Bill answered, again without hesitation, yet with a face exhibiting annoyance.

"So she cannot accuse you of battery of any type?" Larry persisted.

"No, I have not laid a hand on her, not even when we got into an argument...I'm sure you wouldn't be surprised if I said I resented this line of questioning."

"Oh, no, I would be surprised if you weren't resentful. I have only one other question along that line: how frequently do you argue and do you argue in front of the kids?"

"Let me put this way: for the first ten years of our marriage we rarely argued, but since those first years, we have argued more often, and, yes, we argue sometimes in front of the children."

"What do, or what did, you argue about?" Larry asked again.

"Well, some of it is silly stuff—like why didn't you put some gas in the car? But, other stuff had to do with the kids, and, of course, money. With the increase in arguments, there was a decrease in intimacy."

"Good, that's the stuff I need to know about. Now, tell me, has Robin ever earned an honest wage?"

"No, I'm the only wage earner in the family." Bill was rapidly running out of patience and energy to keep up answering the incessant questions. But to his continued annoyance, the questions kept coming.

"So, I assume Robin got an allowance. How frequently did she run over and have to ask for more?"

Right then Bill knew what the term "hot seat" meant. He paused for several moments before he could answer the question. "Well, that's a legitimate question and, as you can imagine, I have had a virtual litany of thoughts and feelings, some of which have to do with physical altercations during heated arguments," Bill answered, knowing Larry would not be satisfied with the answer.

"What do you mean, 'physical altercations'?"

"Are you going to write this down?" Bill asked with some degree of desperation.

"No, I'm not going to write this down."

"I have had mental images where I would get her in a chokehold, but it never went beyond that. I never touched her in a fit of anger. Furthermore, I have.never had thoughts of killing my wife."

"Bill, to me, that is a contradiction. What is the difference between 'mental image' and 'thoughts' of killing your wife? Do you realize that you could be asked that question in some future court action? You'd better decide whether those expression are the same or different," Larry pointed out.

"Yes, I know," Bill responded.

"I went back over your legal documents and, yes, the house is in both of your names. Of course, should one of you pass away, the house automatically goes to the surviving spouse. In your last will and testament, should one of you die before the other one, your assets go to the surviving spouse, also. There is a stipulation concerning the care of the kids should both of you die at the same time: Robin's mother is designated their caretaker and she becomes the executor of your estate. The will specifically lays out how the assets of the estate are to be distributed to the children when they become twenty-six years old," Larry summarized the documents.

"Let me ask you: does the last will and testament address the possibility of divorce?" Bill asked.

"Yes, it does. In the event of a divorce, the care of the children falls to the spouse who stays with the house. It does not specifically address the issue of visitation privileges of the other spouse, but that is something worked out in the divorce decree," Larry answered, paused, and then asked, "Oh, by the way, do you know who is representing Robin in these proceedings?" Larry asked.

Bill frowned and answered, "No, I don't."

Robin Snnithwick, confused and overwhelmed by conflicting emotions, leaned on her lawyer for support, sage advice, and direction in a tortuous and demanding process of legal maneuvering in the manner of a broken marriage. She had contacted Donald Blackman immediately after her husband, Bill, broke the news she had been followed and discovered to be in an adulterous affair with Jackie Moreland.

"Donald, thank you for seeing me right away," Robin opened the conversation.

"You are certainly welcome. Now, let me ask you a few general questions about your marriage with Bill," Donald came right back to her.

"Fire away. Right now I'm an open book," Robin replied, trying to control her fragile emotions.

"How long have you been married to Bill?" Don asked.

"Fifteen years corning up on November 28," she answered.

"And you have two children from this marriage?"

"Yes: Bill Jr., age twelve, and Catherine, age ten," she relied.

"What do the children know about this?"

"So far, they think we are getting a divorce because I don't love their daddy anymore. I admit I am still sorting through conflicting emotions, and I don't yet know how much more to tell them."

"As I see the problem with your children, chances are pretty good they will hear the sordid details from friends or associates at school. I think you are going to have to tell them the whole story," Donald opined.

"I know," Robin responded in a barely perceptible, tremulous voice.

"OK, moving on: what has transpired between you and Bill this last week?"

"Other than my admission that I was having an affair with Jackie Moreland, there really haven't been significant conversations between Bill and me," Robin explained.

"I take it you are now sleeping apart and avoiding each other," Donald observed.

"Right, I am now sleeping in the spare bedroom," Robin explained.

"Are you looking for a place to live?"

"I'm thinking about it, but I have not made any contacts with rental agencies," she answered.

"I take it there are no legal documents that spell out what would happen if one of you filed for divorce," Donald observed.

Robin responded, "No, there are not."

Donald looked through some notes and asked, "OK, now, has Bill ever threatened you or physically assaulted you, either in the past or recently?"

"Once years ago, after a serious argument about money, Bill grabbed me by the shoulders and shook me," she answered.

"That's it? But surely there have been times when he may have threatened you in a non-physical way," he explored the issue further.

"Well, you know, when both of you are arguing, voices rise, but there are no actual threats that would be interpreted as physical or mental intimidation," she answered, keeping her everpresent emotions under wraps.

"But wouldn't you say that raising you voice during an argument is tantamount to intimidation? Particularly, since the male voice, upon raising it, is more forceful," he continued the discussion, trying to clarify whether or not Bill was in any way threatening or intimidating.

"Yes, now that I think about it, it is—it was—intimidating, but I never felt threatened physically—well, maybe, the time he shook me I might have felt physically threatened," she said, not completely sure of what she was trying to say.

"OK, we'll file that away. It may or may not be something we will use in the weeks and months that go by. Now, tell me about your legal documents, specifically your last will and testament."

"I don't think there are any surprises there: it stipulates that, in the event of one of our deaths, the house, its furnishings and the automobiles will go to the surviving spouse. If the wage earner dies, then the assets including a possible retirement account will also go to the surviving spouse. Should both of us die at the same time, then the assets go into a trust for the surviving children. My mother, Mrs. Bradshaw, becomes the executer of the estate in the event both of us die. She would care for the children until their age reaches twenty-six, when they receive share of the estate. There is other stuff in there, but there are no further stipulations that would draw you attention to them," she summarized the last will and testament.

"Now, is there a prenuptial agreement?"

"No."

"Is there any reference to either spouse requesting a divorce?"

"No."

"OK, that's enough for now. Remember, if this legal business gets to where one or both of you get contentious, then it can result in a court action to settle whatever differences might come up. Let's hope it won't get that far. You put your makeup back on, behave yourself and, for God's sake, stay away from Jackie Moreland."

CHAPTER TWENTY

"Is his last name Blackman?"

The summer continued hot and dry. Afternoon showers were common. Even then, some plants were dying from lack of water. The leaf edges were turning in on the bigger, but viable trees. A countywide restriction on the use of water was instituted. The lawns, even with scheduled watering, became brown and dormant.

As far as the friends and neighbors of the Smithwicks were concerned, life was continuing unabated, and the usual study habits of Bill Jr. and Catherine, so far, had remained at the same level as the year before. The Smithwick family was seemingly free of the tensions that were a constant factor in the everyday life of the Moreland family: their usual study habits had gone "south" in the vernacular of Jackie Moreland. Predictably, it was constantly all pins and needles with Jackie and Caroline—as the old saying goes, it was like walking on eggshells for the both of them.

On the other side, Bill resented and remained mad at the fact that Robin was still in the house and seemingly free of a contrite attitude. His feelings were just short of hatred; he could not carry on a conversation with Robin without becoming short and expressing anger. Robin avoided having anything to say to Bill she knew would set him off on a tirade. The wheels of the legal process moved ever so slowly, and Bill's patience was wearing extremely thin. It really got to him that Robin seemed to him to be acting as if nothing were wrong. Thank God for his dental practice; it got him out of the house and away from Robin.

One Saturday night when the kids were out on a sleepover, neither Bill nor Robin were in the mood to go and hide in their respective rooms—it was a situation that screamed out for a confrontation that had the potential to turn ugly.

Again, she came back with, "Look, my lawyer has told me to stay put, unless things get out of hand and turn ugly." Robin repeated herself for what seemed like the hundredth time.

"OK, look, you make a grocery list and estimate the cost and I'll give you that amount of money," Bill said, for once, remaining calm.

Robin smelled a rat—Bill was acting too nice. She surmised he was acting nice so that there could be no question of him attempting to intimidate her, physically or otherwise. It was also pretty obvious to her that he had somehow gotten wind of the date of the upcoming meeting with the lawyers.

She pointed out, "Bill, you are acting too nice," and asked, "Do you know when we are supposed to meet with our lawyers?"

Bill answered the latter question, "Well, let's us just say a little birdie whispered in my ear that it will be on Friday, the thirteenth of next month."

"Thank you. I'll see if I can verify that with Donald," she said, somewhat relieved the time had come to get on with the separation and divorce.

"I think I know Donald—his last name is Blackman, I believe."

"Yes, we met him at church one Sunday," she answered.

"He seems to be a nice guy, but in the heat of battle you never know, but an entirely different side of him may come out," Bill elaborated further.

Robin responded, "He is a nice guy and he has a thorough understanding of what we are up against." She knew Bill knew he had all the advantage in a lawsuit or whatever legal maneuvering was necessary to bring this situation to a close.

"Well, I guess you know that we are filling for a divorce," Bill advised her, stating the obvious with no malice in his voice. He was confident he was getting the house and kids and he wouldn't have to pay alimony.

"Yes, my lawyer and I anticipated you would file for divorce," Robin added, and, then, anticipating that they might argue over some inane subject, she got up and went to her room with no more than a flip of a hand.

Rejecting sleep, she let her thoughts run wild, and, considering the gravity of the situation—she knew she didn't have any chance of a life with Bill—she sought a way out, and the only way out was in the person of Jackie Moreland. *I'm way out on a limb and somebody is about to cut it off,* she thought to herself. *This calls for desperate action,* she thinks, and *I know I'm not to make contact with Jackie, much less call him, but the way I see it, he is my only choice. He said he loved me, didn't he? Suppose I call him at work one day right at eleven o'clock. Oh Jesus, I must be going crazy. No person in their right mind would attempt to call a former lover when the legal wheels are turning and we are close to a resolution of a domestic dispute. To me the biggest problem is: I don't have any satisfactory future—any way I look, the future is bleak, and without Jackie, completely unknown,* she thought to herself.

Robin didn't sleep much that night, but she felt better in the morning knowing there just might be a way out of the situation. She imagined a conversation with Jackie, saying all the well-rehearsed things that would move him in the right direction.

She was having tunnel vision, imagining only the narrow and most comfortable way out of a complicated situation. To her Jackie was the only answer, and she was confident she could convince him the narrow way was the only way.

CHAPTER TWENTY-ONE

"Nine-eleven Calls"

Sunlight streamed through the office window, giving Dr. Jackie Moreland more than enough light to go over the morning notes. His two patients that day were making progress, and it wouldn't be that long before he would refer them to a psychiatrist for long-term anti-depressant and anti-anxiety medicines. He was wrapping up going over the notes, when his cell phone buzzed. He thought, *Who would be calling me between patients? The only persons who had ever called me at this time were Caroline or Robin.* Since he had been told not to talk to or see Robin, he knew it was Caroline.

"Hello, honey, what's up?" Jackie asked in his normal tone of voice.

"Jackie, it's not Caroline," Robin responded.

"Oh, God, Robin, you sure are taking a big chance calling me here," he said, his voice dropping several octaves.

Robin knew what his response would be and, thus, she said with confidence and conviction, "Honey, I don't know about you, but I am about to go out of my mind waiting for the lawyers to do their thing," she said in a desperate voice.

Jackie felt a sensation he hadn't felt in several days and he thought, *Am I going crazy or is my paramour ready to do the only truly desperate thing I could think of—run away!*

After what seemed like eons, she said, "Jackie, are you there?"

"Yes, baby, I'm here and I want you to know I feel the same way you do about all this." Jackie responded and asked with some trepidation, "Do you have something specific you wanted to talk about?"

"Yes, I do, but I want to talk to you face to face, my hands tied behind my back," she said as she chuckled, but she stopped, knowing this was no laughing matter.

"Wow, I had myself convinced we would never see each other again," Jackie admitted, his voice close to a whisper, and then he added, "but, you know what: if both of us were to be caught, what could they do?" Before she could respond, he added, "Well, I don't know what Caroline would do. Besides talking to her lawyer, what could she do, shoot me? I don't think she would do anything beyond what she has already done."

"Jackie, I know I'm impatient, but could you check with Phyllis and see if we could meet in the office tomorrow at noon?" Robin questioned him with love in her voice.

"Hold on, I'll ask her," Jackie said, as he put the phone down.

He came back in a matter of seconds and announced, "She says she knows we both are completely and absolutely out of our minds, but she added the office would be available tomorrow at noon."

"Jackie, do not let me push you into something you don't want to do. It has the potential to push us both into deep water, and I don't know about you, but the best I can do is dog paddle. I'll tell you what: if I don't hear from you until 11:45, then I know we are on. That way you have close to twenty-four hours to think about what we are about to do," Robin elaborated and finished with, "I love you."

Jackie's cell line clicked off. He took some deep breaths, knowing he was going to do this, but also knowing it was going to be hard as hell to face his secretary and his partner—not to mention his wife, Caroline.

The next day was absolutely dead still—nothing moved but a few birds and squirrels. The sun, breaking through the pines, gave warmth to Robin, who had parked behind the office a few minutes before twelve o'clock. She had on her flowery best: a scooped, sleeveless, light-weight dress that was cut above the knees. She slipped into the building and sat on the daybed. And, to no surprise, she had makeup on and that just added to her beauty.

Already stung once, Jackie parked in the back next to Robin's, cut the engine, and opened and closed the driver's side door with no more than a light click. He was clean-shaved with cologne—his stomach twisted into a tight ball.

Jackie stepped into the room and Robin flew into his arms. After a big, tight hug, they kissed long and passionately. It took their breath away and as they stepped back, they both took long deep breaths.

"I love you, too," he said quietly, almost a whisper.

"Oh, boy, is that nice to hear," Robin said with a sigh.

"God, you are just captivating. You are like a magnet and I am the iron filings," Jackie broke poetic and gasped loudly.

They sat on the daybed, holding hands, the gravity of the situation heavy on both their mind and body.

"As far as you know, we were not followed?" Robin asked, looking longingly and deeply into Jackie's eyes.

"No, I don't think so," Jackie answered.

"Dare I say something about the risks we are taking?" she queried.

"Legally, only our lawyers know the risks we are taking, but for us the question of risks is relative—what we are doing is risky, no doubt, but the alternative, at least to me, is unacceptable," he elaborated.

"Here's the question: What are we willing to give up in order for us to be with each other?" Robin asked and moved closer to Jackie.

She ducked under his arm as he anticipated her move. Her dress came up over her knees and he was momentarily distracted—he suddenly wanted her in a bad way and slipped his hand under her dress.

She knocked his hand away and said, "Oh, no, there will be no sex until we decide if we are going to control our future or allow someone else to do that," Robin said, reluctantly.

"I'm pretty sure I know what the answer is, but I have to ask, If we wait for the legal proceedings to play out, how long before we are free and can control our own destiny?" Jackie asked with reluctance.

"It's not bad for me, but you're the one who is giving up a lucrative practice—well, at least, temporarily," she noted, aware that these were reasonable and logical questions to ask, but what they were about to do was neither reasonable nor logical.

"Look, I've had some thoughts about this. If we wait for the proceedings to play out, what will be the cost in legal fees? Hundreds or thousands of dollars? What will be the cost in alimony and child support? What will be the effect on my practice when my patients hear that I'm having an affair and leaving my wife? What will be the effect on your ability to get a job? Regardless of what the answers are, we would have to move away and start all over. So why not start now?" he elaborated at some length.

"For me the monetary question is a moot one. I'm not going to have the responsibilities that you will have and, thus, the answer for me is easy—I say let's get out now. I admit I'm scared, but I'm not going to let this situation be bigger than either of us," Robin responded, again looking deep into Jackie's eyes, searching for determination and commitment—she saw both and cuddled her head into his shoulder at the angle with his neck.

He held her. At the same time, he looked down at his watch and saw it was twelve-thirty.

"OK," he said, "We've got about twenty minutes. Question number one: Are we going to tell our spouses and our children what we are contemplating doing?"

"No, absolutely not," she answered with conviction.

"I agree," he said and then asked, "What is our mode of travel?"

"By far," she said, "it is the critical question. Going by bus or train is safer than going by a car that would be easily recognized. If we take the bus to who knows where, what do we do for transportation when we decide it's time to get off the bus?"

"To me, it's an easy answer," he continued, "we can't take a car that would be recognized, so we take a bus and, then, when we need a car we rent one. And it's important that we don't keep a rent-a-car too long, because that can be traced from the place we rent it from."

"All right, the bus it is," Robin surmised and then added, "we would have to take a taxi to the bus station."

"That leads us to the money situation," Jackie pointed out and asked, "How much money can we raise without there being questions?"

Robin said, "I have a savings account in my name, so I should be able to close the account without a red flag being raised."

Jackie asked, "How much is in the account?"

"About five thousand dollars."

"I do not have a separate account, but I think I could take out about fifteen hundred dollars without it being detected," Jackie said. He looked at his watch and saw he had to go back to work.

He had already thought through what he would say to Phyllis and his partner—one, he was taking two days off; second, if he was not back in two days he was taking a sabbatical of unknown duration; and third, if he was not back in a reasonable amount of time, say a month, then his partner should not only pick up his patients, but also begin a search for a new partner.

Robin also noticed the time and concluded, "We have to pack light so as to travel as fast as possible: one bag each."

"Let's plan on leaving the day after tomorrow; I'll check the bus schedule and get two tickets—what should be our destination?" Jackie asked as he got up to go.

"Just get two tickets to Nashville, Tennessee—that should give us time to make plans from that point," Robin surmised and added, "It's best to get out of the state of North Carolina."

"I guess you know I have to tell my secretary and my partner that I'm taking a leave of absence. She'll have to reassign my patients as openings come up in my partner's schedule. If I'm not back in two months, he will have to hire a second person to fill in," Jackie said, having already thought about what to do with his practice.

He kissed Robin, held her tight, and turned and went back to work. Both had butterflies in their stomachs, and they would stay there for several days.

In the taxi you could hear a feather drop. Robin and Jackie, both, clinched their teeth and tried to still their run-away hearts. They held hands, tighter than ever, Robin's distinctive nails left indentations in Jackie's palms. It hurt, but he said nothing.

In a whisper Robin asked, "So, do you have some cash to pay the man?"

"Yes, I do. A man traveling with his girl should always have money."

In the parking area the taxi driver stopped the car and threw down the flag. He turned toward the back of the taxi and said with a heavy accent, "That'll be seven dollars."

Jackie paid the driver with a ten spot and reminded him they had a piece of luggage each. Neither Jackie nor Robin, upon receipt of their luggage, looked around—they were determined to appear calm, like they rode the bus all the time. Quickly, they bought two bus tickets to Nashville, Tennessee. It was thirty minutes before the bus left, so they sat down in the waiting room and opened books which each had brought with them.

At the half hour, the ticket master clicked on the sound system and announced, "Ladies and gentlemen, the bus to Nashville and points west is in lane three. When the luggage is on board and the hatches are closed, the bus will leave."

Jackie and Robin boarded the bus and scanned the seats, hoping and praying no one would recognize them. It had occurred to Jackie that it would be safer for them to split up, but Robin squashed that in a heartbeat.

Both of them had gotten haircuts and dyed their hair: Robin had become a blonde and Jackie had become a brunette; both of them stepped lightly and even though they had sunglasses on, they did not take them off. When the lights went down, it took them a few seconds to adjust to the interior darkness. The Greyhound bus was about half-full and most of the riders were near the front. Robin and Jackie had already decided to sit all the way to the back and toward one of the corners.

"Nine-eleven," the dispatcher answered. She noted the call at 8:05 P.M., a Thursday.

"Operator, my name is Caroline Morehead. My husband, Jackie, has gone missing."

"When did you see him last?" the dispatcher asked, her questions part of a missing person's protocol.

Caroline expected the question and answered, "About this time Tuesday, the day before yesterday."

"So, it has been at least twenty-four hours?"

"Yes, operator, it has been twenty-four hours," Caroline responded, her voice cracking, tears coming down her cheeks. She sat down her hands shaking. Of all times, it was raining—Caroline didn't like rain very much, as a child she had been caught in a rain storm and was hit by lightning. She was knocked down, but she remembered little of the event—she just knew she didn't like rain, it made her nervous. Rain, to her, was mean and dark, in addition to being wet.

"OK, Mrs. Moreland, I am going to turn you over to another operator who will ask you a series of questions concerning the whereabouts of your husband," the dispatcher instructed Caroline.

Then, another woman came on the line and asked, "What is your husband's full name?"

"Jackie Moreland, he has no middle name," Caroline said, concentrating on a picture of Jackie near the phone, but she could hardly see, her eyes filling with tears. But she could hear the clickety-clack of the computer keys.

"Home address?"

"439 Overland Drive, Statesville, North Carolina."

"Birthdate?"

"October 31, 1954."

"Place of birth?"

"Statesville, North Carolina."

"Caucasian?"

"Yes."

"Glasses?"

"Only for reading."

"Dark glasses?"

"Yes, but only in bright sunlight."

"What color are the frames?"

"Which set of glasses?"

"The dark ones."

"A mixture of light and dark brown."

"Color of hair?"

"Blond, dirty blond."

"Color of eyes?"

"Hazel with a hint of green."

"Height?"

"Six feet even."

"Weight?"

"One hundred eighty pounds, but his weight can vary five pounds or more."

"Any distinguishing features such as scars, tattoos, or birthmarks?"

"Yes, appendectomy scar and a birthmark on his nose, but over the years he has lost the pigment in the birthmarks making them very difficult to see."

"Any congenital abnormalities?"

"No."

"I assume he has changed clothes, but what was he wearing when you saw him last?"

"Dark blue suit with stripped red tie—his work clothes."

"What does he do for a living?"

"He's a psychologist."

"I presume you called his office. What did his receptionist say?"

"She had not seen him since the day before yesterday. The reason she didn't call his home was because he had said he was taking a couple days off."

"He has a partner?"

"Yes, but he was the first person I called and he said he didn't know why Jackie might be missing."

"Has he done anything unusual recently that has caught your attention?"

"No sex."

"Excuse me. What do you mean, 'no sex'?"

Caroline gasped, but held on and said, "He has shown no interest in sex."

"Does Dr. Moreland have a girlfriend?"

"Not that I know of, but I am suspicious," Caroline said, her voice rising indignantly.

"Finally, have you seen his car?"

"That was the first thing I looked for, and it is in the garage."

"Mrs. Moreland, that's all I have for you now. You do have to go to the police station and file a missing persons report. They have to issue an alert and begin the search for your husband," the questioner said and closed the call.

The telephone operator answered the call, "Nine-eleven."

"My name is Bill Smithwick and my wife, Robin, has gone missing," he announced, sadness choking his usual strong voice.

"What is her full name?"

"Robin Smith Smithwick," Bill answered.

"Mr. Smithwick, I am going to send you over to another operator who will ask you some more questions."

"OK."

The next operator began the questioning with a very professional speaking voice, "What is her home address?"

"Three hundred Northridge Drive."

"Birthdate?"

103

"June sixth, 1954."

"Where was she born?"

"Winston-Salem, North Carolina."

"How long has she been missing?"

"Just over twenty-four hours," Bill answered, his voice breaking up.

"Did you say, 'just over twenty-four hours'?"

"Yes, I did."

"Now, I'm going to ask you to give me a description of your wife," the lady instructed Bill.

"Go ahead, I expected as much."

"What was she wearing the last time you saw her?"

"The last time I saw her, she had on a flowery dress with a scoped neck."

"What kind of shoes did she have on?"

"I don't know, I do not remember seeing her shoes."

"What is her height?"

"About five feet seven inches."

"Weight?"

"The last time I can remember her talking about her weight, she said she was overweight at one hundred and twenty-five pounds."

"The color of her hair?"

"Brown or brunette."

"Eyes?"

"Dark brown."

"Caucasian?"

"Absolutely."

"Mr. Smithwick, I have to ask these questions. You'd be surprised how many times 1 have been given an unexpected answer." The operator began again with the questions, "Does she have any distinguishing features like scars, tattoos, or birthmarks?"

"She had a C-section scar, but no tattoos or birthmarks that I have seen."

"Does she have a job or occupation?"

"No, she was a stay-at-home mom."

"How many children do you have?"

"Two."

"What is the gender and age of the children?"

"One of each, a boy eleven and a girl nine."

"Any unusual activities, particularly within the last week or so?"

"Yes, she admitted having an affair."

"Were you able to identify her paramour?"

"Oh, yes, he was a good friend of ours. His name was Jackie Moreland."

"Excuse me. Did you say Jackie Moreland?" the woman asked, a definite lilt in her voice.

"Yes, I did."

"Well, I don't know if I'm supposed to say this, but Jackie Moreland has been reported missing."

"Oh, God, they've run away. As you can imagine, we were in the middle of discussing the fact they were having an affair, and they had been instructed by the lawyers not to contact each other. Lord, this is incredible," Bill said, obviously shocked.

"I presume you have two cars—either one of them missing?"

"No, I presume they took the bus or the train."

"Mr. Smithwick, you'll have to go to the nearest police station and report your wife missing.

"Will do."

"Good. We shall submit a copy of this interview to the police."

Donald Blackman and Larry Jackson III, the lawyers of Caroline Moreland and Bill Smithwick, called an emergency meeting of the principals involved to consider and discuss the shocking news that both of them had run away without so much as a note. All parties to the meeting were in disbelief; they found it completely beyond all reason. Jackie, father and breadwinner, surely could not have abandoned his family and psychology practice—surely on a lark and surely in the throes of lust, for they had had no time to establish a serious and permanent relationship.

Robin, a mother of two children, had always made it a point to put her family ahead of everything else. Since their actions were inexplicable and it may be months before they were found or "Anything else? No? Then let me give you some background information concerning 'Alienation of Affection and 'Criminal Conversation.' I will refer to them as `A-A' and `C-C.' North Carolina is one of a few states that continue to make `A-A' and `C-C' a basis for a lawsuit and divorce proceedings. There are four criteria that are necessary to prove `A-A':

    1)   You and your spouse are 'happily' married. (In the eyes of the law there is no perfect marriage.)

    2)   This happy marriage was 'alienated' and destroyed by the actions of the offending spouse.

    3)   These acts are considered 'malicious' if they include sexual intercourse.

    4)   This 'malicious' intent 'may or may not' include sexual intercourse.

Note: there may be no evidence that the defendant had any 'malicious' intent to break up the marriage."

"If you win a lawsuit based on 'A-A,' the judge may rule compensatory and punitive awards in the millions, but there is a wide variation in the amount of money awarded. In the meantime, do you want Donald and me to prepare the necessary papers for a lawsuit based on infidelity, alienation of affection, and abandonment? A divorce decree naturally follows a lawsuit."

Caroline and Bill, with reluctance, nodded in consent for both the lawsuit and divorce decree. There was no sense of relief—it was a very sad day.

CHAPTER TWENTY-TWO

"On the road"

Jackie and Robin cuddled in the left corner of the back row of the Greyhound bus. They whispered what is classically called "sweet nothings." These were interrupted by a kiss and/or fondling. It wasn't very long, however, before the smooth ride and the engine noise put them to sleep. There were five short stops on the way to Nashville. The overhead lights woke them at each stopping point. Fortunately, they had the back row to themselves and they took advantage of the dark environment when the bus moved on. After about five hours, the lights came back on and the driver announced they were in Nashville. He made a point to say they were in Tennessee, not North Carolina.

Robin observed, "It's the end of the line for us—now the adventure really begins."

"Right, I hope they have a rent-a-car facility," Jackie added.

After they picked up their luggage and went into the terminal, they immediately saw a Hertz Rent-A-Car station and they went directly there, eager to get out of a very public place. Robin looked neither right nor left, but Jackie scanned the entire terminal. He saw a uniformed security guard standing near the boarding gate, but he saw no person in or out of uniform that was the least bit suspicious for police.

"Good afternoon, may I help you?" the agent asked. She was an attractive black woman in a Hertz uniform.

"Yes, we would like to rent a small inexpensive car of light color and it does not have to be new," Jackie answered, pulling his baseball cap farther down over his eyes.

"No problem, we have a small Chevrolet that is what we call `sand' in color," the agent said.

"Good, we'll take it. Do we have to give our destination?" Jackie asked.

"No, you do not. You can turn the car in at any Hertz location, likely a bus, train terminal, or airport," she responded and added, "You are in the system nation-wide, so you are not hard to find."

Just an observation that Jackie and Robin needed, and that made them nervous, but Jackie realized she was talking about the computer system and not that the car could, or would, be traced continuously.

"So, what I hear you say is that we have unlimited miles before we turn it in," Jackie surmised.

"Absolutely," the agent responded firmly, "just sign this agreement and initial these spaces and you're good to go."

"OK, and thank you," Robin spoke up and asked, "Oh, by the way, do you have a map of Tennessee?"

"Yes, we do, and it's free of charge."

"How much do we owe you?" he asked.

"Credit card or cash?" she asked.

"Cash."

"One hundred dollars down and seven and one half cents per mile," the lady said, and then added, "You have to put the gas in at or above the initial reading."

"Where is the car parked?" Jackie asked.

"It's in slot twenty-one, row 'W' near the back gate."

"Thanks, for everything," Jackie said, as he and Robin turned to go. "Honey, we need to make a plan," he said, as he put his free arm around her.

"Yes, I know, but it is not going to be easy. We need to find jobs for us, and, preferably, within walking distance of where we are staying," she responded, placing her free arm around Jackie's waist.

"Robin, look at the map—the first thing in a good plan is picking out a destination. It seems to me Vanderbilt University would be a good place to start," he said.

"I agree, but don't you need to see if Tennessee will honor your license to practice psychology?" Robin asked.

"Absolutely, as I said before, we need to make an application to practice psychology," Jackie said, an edge to his voice. He then added, "I have to find out where the medical board is located."

"Honey, that's the first time you have spoken to me with an edge to your voice," she observed, placing the ball in Jackie's court.

"Baby, I'm sorry," Jackie said, "but I'm really tired and not thinking very well—boy, could I stand a good night's rest."

"I accept your apology—I knew it was the result of a very tense twenty-four hours," Robin said in an easy voice, and added, "By the way, isn't that our car?"

"Yes, thank God, look up Vanderbilt University on the map, I'll drive," Jackie said.

Robin came right back, saying, "The address for the college is 2201 West End Avenue: take the US One/70 South exit and go about five blocks and look for Hutton Hotel. That looks like a good location, and maybe they'll have underground parking," Robin said.

Finding the Hutton Hotel was easy, except they didn't have underground parking. Jackie drove around the hotel and parked in the back, away from the West End traffic. Was he paranoid? Yes, very paranoid. He could have felt worse, but for the disguise. They checked into room 101 under the false names, Mr. and Mrs. Jack Ferrell—or should one say, "false pretenses." Without coming out of their clothes and without pulling back the comforter, they collapsed onto the bed in each other's arms—asleep in minutes.

CHAPTER TWENTY-THREE

"Gone."

D arren Bain, a Statesville detective, showed his badge to the ticket master in the Statesville Greyhound bus station. A plain-clothes policeman was at his side.

"I'm detective Darren Bain and this is my associate, Clarence Jones. We are on the lookout for a couple who may have taken a bus, the day before yesterday. They would have given false names and probably went across the state line into Tennessee. Were you on duty the early morning hours of that day?"

"Yes, I was," the ticket master responded.

"You may want to check your log that day and refresh your memory," Bain said.

"We did have an early run to Nashville, Tennessee," the ticket master said, as he checked his log, and then asked, "What did they look like?"

"They are Caucasian, an adult man and woman, probably pretending they were married. Their age was somewhere in their forties, and they would have worn dark sunglasses to disguise themselves. I imagine they would not have looked particularly well-healed, probably dressed non-descript, but I would imagine they have still stood out. My best guess is that one was a blonde and the other was a brunette, both with short hair," the detective elaborated.

"Yes, I do remember such a couple and, you know, they looked a little nervous—like they were eager to get on the bus. I'm sure they hated to have to wait for the bus to depart."

Bain asked, "What was the destination for the bus?"

"Nashville, Tennessee. They would have had to change buses in Nashville, if they were going farther west."

"Did they get a ticket for farther west, as you say?" Bain asked again.

"No, they only bought two tickets for Nashville," the ticket master answered.

Bain continued to ask questions, "Now, what names did they give you?"

"The man's name was Jack Ferrell, and the woman's name was Catherine Ferrell."

"Oh, so, they presented themselves as a married couple?"

"Well," the man said, "actually they didn't say one way or another, but I just assumed they were man and wife. I suppose they could have been brother and sister."

"Well, thank you very much, you have been most cooperative. But one other question, did they have any luggage?"

"Honestly, I don't remember, but the log says they had only one carry-on a piece."

"Did you actually see them get on the bus to Nashville?" Clarence Jones inquired.

"No, I did not," the ticket master said, emphatically.

"Thank you again. You have been a great help. Here is my card, which has my cell phone number on it, if you want to contact me. You never know they just might come back through here," Darren Bain said.

"I can tell you I'd be shocked if they did."

"Nashville Police Department," the local dispatcher announced.

"This is Darren Bain, one of the detectives from Statesville, North Carolina."

"Yes, detective, what can I do for you?"

"Our local judge has issued a subpoena for a runaway couple who have traveled by bus to Nashville," Bain said.

"I'll switch you over to the desk of our detective on call," the lady said.

"Detective Johnson," Frank Johnson picked up the phone and identified himself.

"Detective Johnson, this is Detective Bain in Statesville, North Carolina."

"What can I do for you, Detective?"

"We are tracking a runaway unmarried couple who have been subpoenaed to appear in court here in Statesville. They are traveling under the assumed names of Jack and Catherine Ferrell. Their real names are Jackie Moreland and Robin Smithwick. Jackie is the male member of the couple. They are being sued by their respective spouses: Smithwick for 'alienation of affection with criminal conversation,' and divorce decree and Moreland for abandonment and divorce decree. We have tracked them as far as Nashville. They left here on a Greyhound bus with tickets for Nashville—the Nashville in your state. We assume they rented a car and are hunting for a place to stay. They would have arrived there sometime after one P.M. today," Bain explained, pausing for expected questions.

"Can you describe them for me?" Johnson asked.

"Yes, both of them are Caucasian, in their forties. The male is six feet, or a little over, with a weight of one hundred eighty to one hundred ninety pounds. The woman is around five feet eight inches in height and one hundred twenty-five pounds in weight. The ticket master here remembers them: they both wore sunglasses and were attractive, but they were wearing non-descript, very casual clothes. Each of them had a small carry-on piece of luggage.

"We called the Hertz rent-a-car station in Nashville, and the agent there said they rented a small tan Chevrolet hybrid. They asked for a map of Nashville. From the description we got from the Greyhound clerk and the Hertz attendant, they had dyed their hair: the brunette woman was then a blonde, and the blond man was now a brunette. I would guess they would have found a place to stay. It seems unlikely for them to change clothes, but I would imagine they have washed the dye out of their hair.

"Finally, they are not criminals and, as far as I can tell, they are not armed. There have not been any criminal charges against them," Detective Bain summarized.

"OK, I've got it. What's the easiest way to reach you?" Johnson asked.

"The easiest and best way to reach me is to call the Statesville Police Department and have the dispatcher page me. Your dispatcher would have that number on record. Thanks for your help."

The first stop for Detective Johnson was the Hertz rent-a-car at the bus station—he had all the information he needed except the exact date and time they picked up the car.

"Ma'me," Johnson got the agent's attention.

"Yes, sir, may I help you?" she asked.

"I am trying to locate a couple on the lam who rented a car from you. The information I have so far is that they are trying to pass as a married couple, Jack and Catherine Ferrell. I was told they came through here yesterday. Can you confirm that and tell me exactly when they rented the car?"

The agent obtained the sign-in log and thrummed through the previous day's entries, paused and said, "Ah, ha, they rented a tan Chevrolet hybrid at exactly two-ten P.M. yesterday. The car had Tennessee plates, tag number ASK-3347."

"Thank you. Now, did they use a charge card?"

"No, they paid one hundred dollars in cash as a down payment."

Detective Johnson asked one final question, "Did they say or ask for anything else?"

"If I remember correctly, they asked for a map of Tennessee," she answered.

"So," Johnson continued with the questions, "they didn't indicate to you what they were looking for or where they were going ?"

"No, sir. Oh, I forgot, they each had a carry-on, a small suitcase."

"Do you remember the color of each carry-on?"

"No, I don't."

"Thank you, ma'me."

"You are very welcome," the agent said, moving over to wait on another customer.

The detective, Frank Johnson, was working alone the day of the telephone conversation with Detective Bain. The detective unit in Nashville was woefully understaffed, putting them at risk, because they had no sidekick or backup. Johnson was trolling the area around Vanderbilt, knowing there were motels and hotels every few blocks or so. He particularly scoped out the parking lots looking for a small tan Chevrolet with Tennessee license plate ASK-3347. He found the car in the Hutton Hotel parking deck. He confirmed it was the right car when he read the license plate. He was a little uncomfortable, because the description of the couple was not all that specific. He headed for the hotel lobby, maybe he just might see a couple that resembled the description Bain had given him.

Jackie and Robin stepped off the elevator, but he stopped short, put his arm in front of Robin, and pushed her back into the elevator.

"What?" Robin asked, her voice strident.

"Did you see that plain black car with a long rear antenna?"

"No, but what's that to us?"

"Well, it means the local detectives have already found our car. Now, there was only one rider in the car, so I'm guessing either his partner has already gotten into the hotel to check the roster for the Ferrell couple or the detective unit in Nashville is woefully under staffed. If we weren't there before, we are now on the lam without transportation, clothes, or the little necessities of life. Thank goodness we have enough money to get us out of Nashville."

"You mean we can't go back and get our things?" Robin asked, her voice breaking up.

"I'm sorry, honey, but we can't go back to the room. It will be staked out and we'd be arrested," Jackie said, trying to soothe her upset feelings. He added, "We need to get a taxi, go to the train station, and get a ticket out of here—you with me?"

"Yes, you know I am," Robin said emphatically and added, "Just like CSI!"

"Hey, that's my girl!" Jackie exclaimed. "I knew you were not only a 'keeper,' but also a 'trooper.'"

"Well, we'll see just how much I can take—I can take a lot as long as I am with you," Robin responded with optimism.

Detective Johnson went directly to the hotel lobby and found the registration desk.

"May I help you?" asked the attendant.

"Yes, you can. I'm Detective Johnson with the Nashville Police Department, and I am tracking a couple by the name of Ferrell."

"Yes, they checked in last night, room 331."

"Thanks for your help," Johnson said as he turned and headed toward the bank of elevators, but he stopped short, remembering he might need a key to the room. He returned to the registration desk and said, "I may need a key."

"It's our policy in these situations that the attendant at the registration takes a copy of the key and goes with the officer to the room," the attendant explained.

"That's fine. I don't think they are dangerous. We have no evidence of them being armed."

The attendant allowed Johnson to knock on the door, room 331. They could not hear any activity in the room.

"Mr. and Mrs. Ferrell, I'm with the police department and I need to talk to you," Johnson said in a loud and demanding voice.

There was no response—no sounds whatsoever.

"OK, open the door," Johnson gave an order to the attendant.

The couple was not in the bedroom and/or in the bathroom. A large king-sized bed did not appear to have been slept in. Two small pieces of brown luggage were on a nearby sofa. Toiletries were in the bathroom. The way the room looked suggested the couple was coming back.

So, if I had my usual sidekick, we would have been able to stake out the car and the hotel room simultaneously, Johnson thought to himself.

The detective went back into the hotel. No one in the lobby fit the description of the Ferrell couple. He again went to the checkout desk and asked if the clerk could buzz his cell phone, if and when the couple attempted to check out of the room. Now he realized that here was another possibility; the couple may not check out of the room in the usual fashion. They just might leave money for the clerk in the room, and sneak out of the hotel. Johnson seriously doubted they would return to the car. To avoid a criminal charge they just might notify the rent-a-car company that they were leaving the car in the parking lot, thinking the down payment would cover what little use they had made of the car. Down deep, Detective Johnson knew that if he could figure out these various possibilities, the couple on the lam could do so also. Considering how they left the hotel room and how they did not go back to the car, it seemed likely they had to take a taxi to the train station. It is also likely they realized they had been spotted and identified, even with the so-called disguise. If they were really smart, they would realize that the detective would follow them to the train station and so it would be best if they would lay low and wait for the heat to cool off. Finally, the thought came to the detective that they just might go back and take the bus to some other destination. He knew he would have to put out an alert and have all the possible means of travel covered.

Jackie and Robin were in a taxi cab heading toward downtown and the bus station. It was an easy decision to go back to the bus station— Jackie knew the train station would be the first place the police would stake out. He was right. The other thing he had to consider was whether or not the police had enough people to also stake out the bus station. He had to take the risk they did not. Using a cell phone, Jackie called the Hertz rent-a-car and told them he had abandoned the car in the Hutton Hotel parking lot and he was mailing the key back to the unit in Nashville. He also requested that they hold on to whatever money they figured he was due.

Shortly before nine o'clock in the morning, Jackie and Robin were left off at the bus station. They had no idea what bus they would be taking—they just knew they would be taking the next bus out of Nashville.

"May I help you?" the attendant at the bus station asked.

"Yes, we would like two tickets to the destination of the next bus out of Nashville."

"The next bus out of here is destined for Charlotte, North Carolina, and points southeast," the attendant said.

"Does the bus stop in Charleston?" Robin asked.

"Yes, it does and, as a matter of fact, Charleston is the last stop for this bus."

"We'll take two tickets to Charleston, then," Jackie requested and asked, "What time does the bus leave?"

"It leaves at nine-thirty."

"Thank you," Jackie said. He took Robin's hand with one of his and took the tickets in the other.

She said in a whisper, "It looks clear so far. Did you know I have an aunt and uncle in Charleston?"

"No, of course, I didn't know that, but it would be a life saver. Do you know them well?" Jackie asked as they found a seat with a view of the parked buses.

"Yes, fairly well. What would we need of them?" Robin responded with a question.

"We might need a place to stay for a few days while we case the city and find a safe place for us to stay on a more permanent basis," Jackie expounded.

"Ladies and gentlemen, the bus to Charlotte and points southeast is now loading," the attendant announced.

"Well, baby, here we go again," Jackie said, hooking his arm around her waist.

"Don't you think it's pretty amazing we have not had sex for four days?" Robin whispered.

"Don't worry about that. We'll more than make up for the days we've missed—it will just make it better, if that's possible," Jackie replied in a quiet voice.

"You know that's what I love about you: you are the eternal optimist," she observed, again in a voice meant only for her lover.

"It is only because of you that I am such an optimist. And speaking of days without sex, we are looking at another exhausting trip and the need to rest," he said, taking her arm to get on the bus.

Once again the couple sat close together in the left back corner of the bus. When the lights went down, they cuddled and whispered sweet nothings as before. As the bus hit its rhythm, they slowly slacked off the cuddling and finally went to sleep.

CHAPTER TWENTY-FOUR

"At long last they stopped running"

Detective Johnson knew he was losing track of the runaway couple. No, they did not take the train: the ticket master told Johnson he had no such persons on the train that was to stop in Nashville that morning. Johnson checked once again the Hutton Hotel and found no evidence that the couple had come back to claim their personal items—the rent-a-car was in the same spot as before. He found out that the Hertz Company had been made aware of the fact that one of their cars had been abandoned. Johnson felt a little silly and stupid when he went back to the bus station and found out the runaways had boarded a bus for Charlotte, North Carolina, with a final destination of Charleston, South Carolina.

Since the trip from Nashville to Charlotte took nearly four hours, Jackie knew the police or a detective would be waiting for them in Charlotte. That meant they had to get off the bus at the stop just before Charlotte, which would be Gastonia. The only logical choice they had was to somehow get a ride from Gastonia to Greenville, South Carolina, where they could get back on the bus, knowing the North Carolina police would have no jurisdiction in South Carolina.

The only way, it seemed to Jackie, they could avoid the police and get to Greenville was to hitchhike down interstate eighty-five.

Jackie felt like they would be able to get to the Greenville bus station in time, if they had luck on the interstate. But Robin had a better idea: rent a car in Gastonia and drive to Greenville and re-board the bus to Charleston. If the couple did not get off the bus in Charlotte, they realized the North Carolina authorities would notify the South Carolina police in Greenville. Knowing that "alienation of affection" and "divorce decree" and abandonment were not criminal charges, there was a chance the South Carolina police would not apprehend the North Carolina couple. In addition to "alienation of affection" not being a criminal offense, it was also not recognized in the state of South Carolina as a reason to start divorce proceedings.

So the couple got off the bus in Gastonia, rented a car, and drove to Greenville, across the border between the two states. No police were to be seen at the bus station and the bus driver recognized their ticket to Charleston. With a great sigh of relief, they got back on the bus and rode all the way to Charleston, sleeping most of the way.

It was late in the evening when the bus got to Charleston. Even with what sleep they got, Jackie and Robin were tired and sore, but were glad to see the dark sky that would cover their movements. As far as they could tell, there were no police or other peace officers waiting for them. They could not count on being free of the authorities—every movement had to be calculated to keep them out of the clutches of the police. If there was any way to plan their activities two or three times in advance, the safer they were going to be.

So the first move was to get in touch with Robin's aunt and uncle to see if they could put them up for a few days.

Jackie asked Robin, "Do you know your aunt's phone number or address?"

"No, I don't, but I'm sure they are listed in the phone book," she replied and added, "since we have to go to the drug store for needed necessities, we can call them from there. It is a nice convenience they are 'William and Stacy Smithwick.'"

Uncle William answered the phone on the fourth ring, "Hello."

"Uncle William, this is Robin."

"Well, my goodness, what in the world you doing in Charleston?" he asked.

"It's a long story, Uncle William, and I'll tell you all about it when I see you," Robin replied.

"Where are you?"

"We're at the CVS near the bus station."

"That's easy, we're not that far from you," her uncle said and added, "tell you what, let me pick you up, I assume you don't have a car—did you say, 'we'?"

"That would be great...you are right, we don't have a car and, yes, I said 'we.' I am traveling with a man named Jackie Moreland."

"I'll be there in five minutes to pick the both of you up," her uncle said and he hung up.

The Smithwicks lived on Meeting Street in downtown Charleston in an apartment over a business establishment. True to his word, her uncle was at the CVS pharmacy in five minutes.

"Uncle William, this is Jackie Moreland, a dear friend of mine," Robin said.

"Jackie, it is nice to meet you—any friend of Robin's is a friend of mine. I presume you guys will tell me why you have no luggage," Uncle William said, stating the obvious.

"Oh, yes, we'll tell you why we have no luggage; it's part of a very long story."

He responded, predictably, "You pop up at the bus station, you have no car and no luggage, and you have a 'dear friend' who is not your husband. I'll bet, in addition to it being a long story, it is also a complicated and interesting story...am I right?"

"Yes, sir, you are right. When the story is done, we'll have to talk about whether or not it would be prudent to call the Smithwicks in Statesville," Robin said, aware of the consequences they would have to face.

"Oh, boy, this sounds like it could be a romantic novel, but, even with that, we'll have to do what is right," her uncle said, speaking like an uncle.

"That's what I thought you would say, but, when you hear the story it may not be so prudent to call home."

"You mean the prudent way may not be the right way," her uncle said sternly.

"Yes, but when we look at all sides of the picture, it may be difficult to make the right decision," Robin said, adding, "I'm not sure we can discern what is right or wrong in the case—it is simply one decision in a whole array of decisions that have already been made."

"I can see that...I'm sure you've already made a whole host of decisions before you came to this point. Remember, it's a brother you're talking about."

"Well, here we are. I'm sure your aunt Stacy will have a lot to say about this," Uncle Bill spoke, trying to bring the conversation to a close.

Stacy Smithwick, like her close-to-the-vest personality, kept a very neat house. In her world, there was no such thing as an unexpected surprise; she simply stayed prepared for the unexpected and that included how she dressed and how she presented herself. When she saw Robin, crumbly from the long trip, and a strange man, equally crumbly, she knew right away this was going to be bad news. As a matter of fact, she suspected from the get-go this was likely the result of an affair. It made her sick to her stomach, and she prayed this was not what it appeared to be.

Robin, Jackie, and Uncle William came into the great room of the Charleston Smithwick's apartment. The two vagabonds waited for the inevitable thunder that was Stacy when she was aroused, particularly when she perceived a wrong has been committed. But before Stacy jumped to any conclusions, she hugged her niece and shook Jackie's hand.

"My God, what have you two done?" Stacy asked, a tone of righteous indignation in her voice. "Robin, I want to hear from you first."

"Aunt Stacy, we have done our families a great wrong—Jackie and I are not only involved in an illicit love affair, but we have also run away from home. It won't cut much ice, but we are in love and plan on staying together."

"The illicit love affair I can surely see, but why did you not go through the proper channels and settle this among the lawyers or in court before you ran away. Surely you know you've done yourselves a gross injustice," Stacy observed in a logical line of thought.

"We have no logical explanation for our actions, Aunt Stacy," Robin said, just short of tears.

"Well, first of all, you have to call home, both of you," Stacy said, firmly.

"I'll go first," Robin said softly, tears in her eyes.

"Hello," Bill answered the phone, home for the weekend.

"Bill, this is Robin," she was having trouble making even medium-length sentences.

"Robin, where are you? We have been beside ourselves with worry; you know, of course, the police have put out an alert for your whereabouts," Bill said, both surprised and earnest.

"We're in Charleston with Uncle William and Aunt Stacy," Robin answered.

"It's obvious for me to ask: when, if ever, are you coming home?"

"Bill, I don't know how to answer that question, but right now we are going to start a new life together, so the best answer is not right away," Robin answered, the tears now wetting her cheeks.

"Well, as far as the law is concerned, we have a year's separation to make up our minds. But, for me, the trauma you have served on us is way too much for reconciliation," Bill said and then added, "I'm trying to approach this in a calm, cool, and collected fashion, but unless you come home right now, I see no chance for us, and especially for the kids."

"Bill, you do what you have to do, but I am not coming home right away. Having said that, is there any way I could talk to the kids?" Robin said—for some reason she had to ask—knowing there was probably no chance she could talk to the kids.

"Look, Robin, there is no way I can make any reasonable decision about the kids—let me think about it. Will Uncle William and Aunt Stacy know where you are?" Bill asked.

"As long as we are under their roof, you are free to call. Otherwise, I'm not going to put that kind of risk on my aunt and uncle. If somebody were to inquire as to our whereabouts, William and Stacy will have to say they don't know and they will be speaking the truth," Robin explained.

"OK, well, this is goodbye," Bill said bluntly.

"All right, Jackie, it's your turn," Stacy said.

"Hello," Caroline answered the phone—she had no idea who might be calling.

"Caroline, this is Jackie."

"Jackie, where in the world are you and do you plan on coming home any time soon?" Caroline asked, desperation in her voice.

"Caroline, right now Robin and I are in Charleston with her aunt and uncle," Jackie said softly and added, "Right now we are not going anywhere else. We are hoping to find a place to stay here."

Caroline broke down and sobbed, "Well, we are officially separated, and you will be served divorce papers."

"I realize that and I'm sorry it has to happen this way. I know it would be inappropriate for me to speak to the kids under these circumstances, so if they ask about me tell them I am all right and living in Charleston and maybe, someday, we'll be able to see each other."

"OK, but you let me know how to get in touch with you—you never know, the kids may want to talk to you," Caroline said, seemingly calm, but not completely collected.

"It would be best to call me on my cellphone, 919-312-5467, because I have no idea where we will finally settle down," Jackie said and closed the line.

"Well, you two, you may stay here until you find a place to stay on your own," Stacy concluded.

"Aunt Stacy, I appreciate what you are doing. We won't stay any longer than we have to," Robin said with sincerity.

"Robin, let me say something obvious: you and Jackie have broken the laws of God, and it is up to God to forgive you. William and I will pray for the strength to forgive you, also," Stacy said in conclusion.

"Thank you for your forthrightness, we know what we have done and we will carry it to our grave," Robin said and added, "We need to get some rest. Where do you want us to bed down?"

"Robin, you and Jackie cannot sleep together in my house, and, fortunately, we have two available bedrooms and I will show you where to sleep," Stacy said with authority,

There was a bone-deep sadness in the Moreland household, a sadness that produced a terrible quietude which was persuasive and yet, at the same time, the smallest noise jolting to any and all. The children walked around in a daze, frequently bumping into furniture and doorjambs. It was eerie, nearly as quiet and weird as a death in the family. Somehow, Caroline held it together in front of the children, but, at night, in Bill's and her bed, she cried herself to sleep. The children weren't totally out of it—they could tell when she had been crying.

Now, in the Smithwick home, anger was the mood of the day. Bill couldn't believe Robin had deserted him and the children. His anger masked his underlying feeling of sadness and remorse. Would Bill have taken Robin back? Yes, certainly, but it would have to be conditional. Robin would have to make the contact, express a sincere contriteness, and be prepared for a certain amount of hurt in the children. But it was not to be—somewhere, somehow the relationship had crossed the Rubicon and there was no turning back.

"Honey!" Jackie whispered, appearing in the dark room like a spirit from another time and place.

"What? God, I thought you were a ghost—damn, Jackie, you know what Stacy said, we can't sleep together," Robin woke from a sleep filled with strange apparitions.

"Well, I'm sorry, but we are consenting adults, and she can't tell us what we can and can't do or how we are to live our lives," Jackie said with conviction.

"OK, I know how you feel and I feel the same way, but if we do this, we can't have sex," Robin whispered.

"Oh, shit, Robin, how will she ever know what went on in here?" he asked, irritated.

"Jackie, I don't want to be put into a situation that calls for a lie," she said, a tone that Jackie knew she was not going to allow him to have sex with her.

"OK, move over and we can cuddle until we go back to sleep. She'll probably catch us in the morning no matter what we do," he responded, a resigning aspect to his voice.

"All right, but no petting."

"I figured that out, but you are going to owe me, babe…I can store just so much love in this poor body of mine."

They cuddled until they went back to sleep, but there was no groping. Fortunately, they both woke up shortly before Stacy did and Jackie went back to his room, walking on his tiptoes, quiet as a mouse, but, as it turns out, he was unable to fool Stacy.

"Good morning, you two," Stacy, looking at them both, added, "I found an empty bed last night."

Jackie was ready for the challenge, "Yes, I'm to blame, but, for what it's worth, we behaved ourselves."

"OK, I'll take that at face value, but you know sleeping together is for married couples," Stacy said, telling them something they already knew, but making sure they had an appropriate amount of guilt.

"Guilty as charged," Jackie said, some resentment in his voice.

"OK, breakfast is just about ready. What are you two going to do today?"

"The first thing we have to do is to rent a car and then we have to find a place to stay," Robin answered her question.

"Well, I'm not sure where the closest place is to get a car, but there are rooms, small apartments, and bed and breakfasts up and down Meeting Street and its many crossing streets," Uncle William said, jumping into the conversation and breaking a long period of silence. He added, "If someone calls here asking for one of you, what are we supposed to say?"

Jackie took his question and said, "First of all, ask them to identify themselves and to tell you what their relationship is to either one of us. If they are family, take a number and tell them we'll call back," and then she added, "If they are the police or other authorities, do not lie, just tell them we are not here."

"On that note, let me change the subject," Jackie said and asked, "What do you have for a headache?"

"Aspirin or Advil? How bad is it?" Stacy asked.

"Oh, not too bad, so I don't think it matters, but I will go with a couple of Advil's," Jackie answered, rubbing his right temple area.

Stacy opened up a bottle of Advil and gave two tablets to Jackie. He thanked her and they settled down for a breakfast of eggs, bacon, and toast.

Jackie and Robin walked up and down Meeting Street. Most of the buildings that fronted the street were businesses, but the crossing streets had bed and breakfast facilities and they took the first one they came to. Fortunately, the weather was cooperating: it was sunny and warm.

Jackie asked the attendant at the bed and breakfast, "Can you tell me where the nearest Hertz or Avis car rental unit is located?"

"The only car rental places that I know of are at the airport," the attendant answered.

"That means we'll have to take a taxi to the airport," Jackie said and asked, "If you don't mind, would you call a cab for us?"

"I'll be glad to—just wait outside and I'll have a cab pick you up."

The cab was at the bed and breakfast in ten minutes, and the driver asked them where they needed to go.

Jackie responded to the driver, "We need to go to the nearest Hertz or Avis rent-a-car unit."

"Well," the driver turned and said, "I'll have to take you to the airport."

Jackie had heard that so many times, he was beginning to think there was a conspiracy.

"How much is the fare?" Robin asked.

"Ten dollars, city-wide," the driver answered quickly, and then asked, "Do you still want me to take you there?"

"Yes, please," both Jackie and Robin answered quickly and then laughed at each other.

After they picked up a car, both knew the first stop they were going to make was the bed and breakfast.

"Honey," Robin asked Jackie, "how is your head?"

"It's throbbing a little, but it's not bad as it was, thanks to the Advil," Jackie answered and added, "Maybe we can catch a nap and see if the throbbing goes away."

"I'm hoping that's not all we'll catch," Robin said with a chuckle.

Fifteen minutes to the airport, ten minutes to rent a Ford Fusion, and fifteen minutes to drive back to the bed and breakfast. Right away parking became a problem and they had to park three blocks over, but nothing was going to quiet their anticipation that they would soon be alone with no concern for the time of day. Finally, at long last they had a place to lay their heads—real or not, they felt a sense of security. Neither had the energy or desire for sex—they crashed onto the bed and were asleep in minutes.

CHAPTER TWENTY-FIVE

"I don't want him back"

Bill Smithwick was beside himself—the truth was coming at him from a multitude of directions. Not only had Robin gone, but she had run away without a goodbye. The children were also beside themselves. What on earth would have caused mother to run away with a close friend's husband? Life was tough enough without the disappearance of the very person you loved the most.

Bill was not going to take this abrupt absence of his wife lying down. Right or wrong, he was going to find Robin and get some answers—maybe even scare her a little bit, her just reward for abandoning her family. With no hesitation, he called Frank Johnson.

"Frank, this is Bill Smithwick."

"What's up, Bill?"

"You've probably heard about Robin and Jackie Moreland running away," Bill responded.

"Oh, yes, I heard about that a few days ago," Frank replied.

"Frank, I've been mad at them ever since, and I can't let this thing die! What are my options?"

"Bill, I understand the police have been chasing them, but they are now in South Carolina, out of the police's jurisdiction."

"Yes, I know, and it just makes me more frustrated by the minute.

We did get a phone call from Robin. She was with her aunt and uncle in Charleston—her Aunt Stacy is not happy with the situation, but there is not a lot she can do, because of loyalty to Robin. Her aunt is an upstanding Christian woman and she would not tolerate this kind of behavior. But, at the same time, she is the kind of person who would give her niece the benefit of the doubt. One thing I do know, however, she would forbid them from having sex in her home. I'm sure they will find a place all their own, allowing them freedom to do whatever they want. And that brings up another thing: they were barely more than friends—how can they be in such heat?" Bill concluded—many questions, few answers.

"Bill, think about it. They certainly are in heat and maybe it's because everything is so new. So, first of all, we have to find out where they are staying. Do you think her aunt and uncle would tell us where they are?" Frank asked.

"No, I think her aunt is savvy enough she would not want to know where they are—that way she'd tell no lies," Bill responded.

"You're probably right, but since they were the last person to see Robin, we have to start with them," Frank said, definitively.

"I'll get the telephone number in Charleston for her aunt and uncle. Are you going to make the call and what are you going to say?" Bill inquired.

"Yes, I'll make the call and I'm going to say you have hired me to track them down and bring them home. I'll ask Stacy if she has any idea where they are," Frank said.

"If we do find them, you know they'll say they are not coming home. There is nothing but trouble for them in North Carolina—starting with a lawsuit and divorce decrees," Bill elaborated.

"I think we have to scare them into thinking we will kidnap them and bring them back to this state," Frank said with conviction.

"I think we can scare them without threatening them, Frank," Bill countered.

"OK, let's brainstorm and come up with something less threatening," Frank acquiesced and added, "What, then for them is the most important thing?"

"That's easy: as much as I hate to say it, the most important thing for them is each other," Bill said.

"OK, we have to create a scenario that would separate them, sending one of them home," Frank observed.

"I agree. That's a start, but we will need the services of a lawyer," Bill noted and added, "I'll contact my lawyer and see what our options are—we may have to include Caroline Moreland in this discussion."

Bill called Larry Jackson the Third.

"Larry Jackson," he answered, picking up his ownline.

"Larry, Bill Smithwick."

"Hey, Bill, what can I do for you?" Larry asked.

"I'm working with Frank Johnson and we're trying to get Jackie Moreland and my wife, Robin, home from Charleston, South Carolina, where they, at least for now, are staying with Robin's aunt and uncle, William and Stacy Smithwick. To our knowledge they have had no contact with the police or other authorities. We are looking at the possibility that they'll come home if we can separate them. We thought we could make that happen if you can come up with a plan based on a difference in the implementation of the law as it applies to one or the other. I would think Robin is the more vulnerable of the two and a charge of abandonment might put the pressure on her to come home, particularly if we say the charge might be dropped if she cooperates and rejoins her family," Bill summarized.

"Bill, I hate to be so blunt, but you are whistling in the wind. Those two know what the score is, and they are not about to separate and allow one of them to come home and face the music. Look, they made the decision to run away together, they think they are in love, and the sexual tension, I imagine, is quite high. For whatever reason, they have decided this new relationship is more important than their family relationships they voluntarily left behind," Larry stated in no uncertain terms.

"Larry, I'm sure you are right, we are whistling in the wind, but we hoped maybe you had an idea that might put the pressure on them to come home," Bill replied, a noted drop in tone of voice.

"Look, you face the music: they don't want to come home. Again, to be blunt, you are 'sucking the proverbial hind tit,'" Larry brought the hammer down, hoping to get Bill to see the situation for what it really was. To Larry the die had been cast and Bill and Caroline and their children would have to start over.

"All right, I read you loud and clear. I'll get with Caroline and see if she wants to pursue this any further, maybe try another lawyer," Bill closed and phoned Caroline immediately.

"Caroline, Bill Smithwick."

"Oh, hey Bill, what's up?"

"Caroline, I've been talking with Frank Johnson, a free-lance operative who intervenes into situations like you and I are experiencing, and to Larry Jackson, my lawyer. They, particularly Larry, don't see where we have any chance of getting Jackie and Robin to come home. Larry questions why we would want them back after they have essentially ruined their marriages and crushed the lives and hopes of their kids. Would you want to contact a different lawyer and see if there is any way we coiuld put pressure on them to come home?"

"Bill, I'm still grieving, but I'm past the point where I would welcome Jackie back home. The children and I are undergoing psychotherapy, and it's going better than I anticipated. I realize now we can get on with our lives without Jackie. I am getting to the point where I can wish them well and I just don't think we can, or want to, start over," Caroline expounded on the fact she saw the relationship was beyond repair.

"Caroline, I can understand where you are coming from, and I am glad to hear you are making progress to get on with your lives. Let's get the kids together—that should help all of us to move on," Bill said, relieved to know the reaction to the affair and abandonment had taken a positive turn toward recovery.

"I'm not sure getting the kids together would help us move on, but that is my basic pessimistic nature. I'll tell you what: I will think about your suggestion and maybe even talk to the kids and get back to you. One thing I would like to do is for you and me to have dinner away from the children," Caroline responded, showing she could make a positive suggestion.

"All right, Caroline, I'll wait for your call—I would love to go out to eat with you. Goodbye, for now," Bill replied, also in a positive manner.

Jackie and Robin now had a way to get around and a place to stay. After a visit to the pharmacy, they returned to the bed and breakfast. After so many hours of nervous paranoia, they finally paused, took a deep breath, and settled down to just be with each other. They threw the covers on the bed back, took their clothes off, collapsed into each other's arms and kissed long, hard, and deep. Slowly they made extremely passionate love.

"That was wonderful, fantastic and, like art, beautiful to the extreme," Robin in a whisper waxed poetic, her eyes closed.

Jackie responded in kind, "All I know is it was utterly and absolutely out of this world. I have to say it was surely meant for us to be together and to share these incredible feelings—love, love, and more love."

"I agree," Robin cooed and added, "It was probably a degree of selfishness out of the ordinary, an ego trip of the first order."

"Well, all I can say is we experienced a power beyond the ordinary, a sensation above the natural, an otherworldly state seemingly unreachable in the here and now," Jackie expounded and then added, "Robin, this is crazy talk. We sound like a pair of parrots, talking out of our gourd. Let's just say it was wonderful and, after cleaning up, go get something to eat," Jackie said and then with a frown on his face added, "I've got another headache, worse than the other one."

"Honey, take some medicine and if that doesn't help, we'll have to go see a doctor. It's not lost on me that there are some very real drawbacks to going to a city where we have no connections and no one to advise us on things such as our health," Robin decreed, suddenly down to earth.

"Boy, you are a killjoy—what happened to all the passion?" Jackie asked with a chuckle, and then flipped the top off a bottle of Tylenol.

"Well, I guess one of us has to keep us grounded and, no kidding, we have to take care of ourselves. Let's not drive to dinner—just leave the car unlocked and rigged so that we can determine whether or not someone has been in the car," Robin replied, speaking like she was a detective. She added, "OK, I'll shower first and make up the bed. You know we are going to have to buy some clothes, particularly since we're not far from winter."

"You're right on all counts...I can see why I love you so much. Incidentally, I'm sure our families know where we are. Don't you think we should try to reach the kids? I'd love to hear their voices," Jackie said, the latter part with a lilt in his voice.

Robin frowned and sighed, "Honey, I'm not sure that's a good idea. However, it might be a good idea to call our folks and let them know we are alive. Let's discuss all of this at dinner. Looking at the brochure we got from the landlady, there's a nice restaurant within walking distance. I'm going to clean up and, as Kris Kristofferson says, I'm going to put on my 'cleanest dirty shirt.'"

"Robin, the name of the restaurant is the same as the address: 'Eighty-two Queen.' It is supposed to have some of the best crabcakes in the world, and that makes my decision real easy as to what I am going to eat, and it is just a few blocks down Meeting Street."

"Sounds good to me...I love crabcakes," Robin responded.

Besides their frumpy clothes, they continued wearing hats and sunglasses just in case somebody might be in Charleston looking for them. They were not about to make any slipups, if they could help it.

CHAPTER TWENTY-SIX

"Solo lawyer/Detective Jake Lambert"

Frank Johnson got word from a local detective that the two run-aways were in Charleston, South Carolina, staying with Robin's aunt and uncle, William and Stacy Smithwick. Frank knew a solo lawyer/detective in Charleston, Jake Lambert. He called him.

Answering the first ring, coffee in hand, Jake said, "Hello, this is Jake Lambert."

"Jake, Frank Johnson in Statesville, North Carolina." Frank had known him for years, having met him at one of the national meetings for detectives.

"Frank, it seems like it's been years since I talked to you. I haven't seen you since one of our meetings years ago. What's going on?" Jake asked.

"Well, the truth of the matter is I haven't been going to the meetings for one reason or another. Jake, I have been hired to track down a wayward unmarried couple who are apparently in lust, maybe truly in love, and they have gotten down to your neck of the woods. Their names are Robin Smithwick and Jackie Moreland. They are traveling under assumed names: Mr. and Mrs. Jack Ferrell.

"The paperwork is in progress, but it looks like they are going to be charged with 'alienation of affection' and a lawsuit based on abandonment. There are no criminal charges. They are, or were, staying with Robin's aunt and uncle, a Mr. and Mrs. William Smithwick. I don't have their phone number or address, but I understand they are listed in the phone book. Would you contact their aunt and uncle and find out as much as you can about their niece and her paramour? I don't know how much we can do about this situation, but their families are interested in knowing where they are, what they are doing, and what laws they have broken, if any. I'll split the fee with you," Frank explained.

"I'll take it from here. While you were talking, I found the aunt and uncle in the phone book—they live on Meeting Street. If their niece has moved on, I think it would be better for me to call on them personally. You know the routine: it's easier to tell if they are lying by speaking with them face to face. I'll go out there this evening in case one or both of them are working," Jake said with confidence in his voice. Things had been a little slow for him, and this was just the kind of assignment that he would find interesting.

He added, "You take care and I'll be in touch, hopefully sooner rather than later."

"Thanks, Jake, I appreciate this," Frank said as he closed the call.

Jake found the address easily and rang the bell to the Smithwick's apartment. Uncle William answered the door. He appeared to be just home from work: his tie was undone and his jacket was off.

"Yes, what can I do for you?" he questioned the stranger, who was in a dark turtle-neck sweater and brown jacket.

"Is this the Smithwick home?" Jake asked.

"Yes, it is," William answered.

"My name is Jake Lambert, and I am a free-lance detective. I have been contacted by a detective in Statesville, North Carolina, concerning the whereabouts of a couple on the lam, a Robin Smithwick and a Jackie Moreland. I understand you may know where they are now staying. I'd like to talk to them—I'll be no threat to them."

"Mr. Lambert, they were here the last couple of days, but they have moved on and I don't know where they are staying," William said, exhibiting a clear-cut honest demeanor.

"Were they in an automobile?" Jake asked, sensing that this man was being honest about the whereabouts of his niece.

"No, they took a cab," William responded.

"Can you tell me what they were wearing?" Jake asked.

"Yes, both of them were in very casual clothes, and it looked like they had been sleeping in them. She was in a non-descript tan blouse and brown skirt; he was in a wrinkled white dress shirt and grey slacks," William answered.

"Mr. Smtihwick, would your wife know any more than you do about where they might have gone?" Jake persisted with another question.

"Well, I'll let you speak to my wife. Honey, will you come to the front door?"

"Yes, William, what do you need?" Stacy asked, as she came to the front door.

"This is Detective Lambert, and he is looking for Robin and Jackie," Uncle William explained.

"I'm sorry, but I can't help you. They left here in a cab yesterday without so much as a goodbye," she explained, unable to mask her impatience.

Jake could see they had no idea where their niece had gone to, but if anyone were covering for the pair, it would be Stacy Smithwick. He observed once again, "Your husband tells me they had no luggage. I find that quite unusual for someone traveling in a large city."

William spoke up, "I agree with you. I thought it was very unusual for a pair of travelers to be without luggage, unless, of course, they had to get out of Nashville, Tennessee, in a hurry. As I understand it, they went by bus through Charlotte and Greenville. Have they broken any laws?"

"I don't think they have broken any federal or South Carolina laws," Jake answered.

"Well, Mr. Lambert, I'll be blunt with you," Stacy said with her usual forcefulness, "if I knew where they were or where their luggage was, I wouldn't tell you. They certainly don't fall into your bailiwick and I agree with you, I don't think they have broken any laws of this state, either."

"Well, OK, that's fine—I know how you feel and I won't bother you anymore," Jake replied and turned and walked toward his car, but not before saying, "Look, if the situation does call for someone of my 'bailiwick' as you call it, please consider letting me know. I mean them no harm."

"As the kids say all the time, 'fat chance,'" Stacy said in a voice he was sure to hear loud and clear.

Jake called Frank Johnson back and said, "Well, I got to talk to the Smithwicks and they didn't know anything about the whereabouts of their niece, and I believe them. And, they said with emphasis that if they knew where she was, they wouldn't have told me and I believe them on that, too."

Frank was a little disappointed, but he wasn't surprised they were not going to be cooperative, and he said, "I'm not surprised, Jake."

Jake quickly added, "Frank, there is one thing I think should be checked out: they left the Smithwicks in a cab. So one of the first things they might do is to rent a car. Let me talk to the Hertz and Avis people at the airport and see if a Mr. and Mrs. Jack Ferrell rented a car."

"That's a good idea—they have previously rented a car, so they would likely do the same thing in Charleston," Frank said.

Jake drove to the airport, parked, and walked up to the Hertz attendant and said, "I have been hired to find a Mr. and Mrs. Jack Ferrell, who might have rented a car yesterday. Can you help me?"

"I might be able to," responded the attendant, "Just let me check my log." The attendant broke out a bound volume and leafed through the most recent entries and said, "Yes, I have an entry for a Mr. and Mrs. Jack Ferrell. They rented a late-model white Ford Fusion."

"Good, do you have a license plate number?" Jake asked.

"Yes, it's South Carolina tag number: FED-3999," the attendant answered.

"Thank you, I appreciate your cooperation," he said, as he offered her a ten spot for her trouble.

She politely declined the ten spot and said, "That was completely unnecessary...you have offended me and you will get no more cooperation."

Jake called Frank a second time and told him what he had found out about the recent movements of the run-away couple operating under false pretenses. He now had knowledge of the car they had rented.

"Frank, I will put out an alert for that car with those South Carolina plates," Jake said and added, "1 don't think it will take more than a day or two to find the car and possibly the occupants."

"Jake, you had better be careful...to my knowledge they have not broken any laws of this state," Frank said, raising a caution flag. Then he added, "We could face a lawsuit for unlawful abridgement of a citizen's rights."

"So, are you telling me to call off the alert?"

"I'll tell you what: I'm going to drive down to Charleston and should be there sometime tonight. So just hold off on the alert until I get there, and we'll put our heads together and come up with a plan that's lawful. Is your office still next to the Charleston administration building?" he asked.

"Yes, it is and I will be on my cell numbered 843-304-9697," Jake answered.

"I'll buzz you when I get into town," Frank replied and signed off.

Jackie and Robin enjoyed the crabcakes at "Eighty-two Queen." They walked the few blocks back to their bed and breakfast, having an animated conversation about the rent-a-car.

"Honey, we were lucky to find a parking garage near where we are staying and where we could keep an eye on the car. Now I don't think we need to drive it unless we absolutely have to. It would be easy enough to get a description of that car from the Hertz people. It is likely that Bill or Caroline or both hired a private detective to find us. So, the question would have to be: did the detective get a description of the car and have the Charleston police sent out an alert stating that the occupants of the car are wanted for questioning?" Jackie expounded.

Robin put her CSI hat on and said, "Jackie, I'm not sure a lawyer or a detective could justify impounding that car and questioning its occupants. We are not criminals, and it would be easy for the South Carolina authorities to overstep their bounds and be guilty of a citizen's rights violation."

"Hey, you've got a good point there...I hadn't thought of it that way. You know, considering what we've done, it's easy to begin feeling guilty about this whole mess. Let's get a good night's rest and re-think this tomorrow."

After a restless night with intermittent sleep, but with a solid breakfast, Jackie and Robin first checked on the rent-a-car and found nothing unusual—there was no evidence that anybody had done anything more than just look into the car. They replaced the small piece of paper that was in the left front doorjamb. Deciding to make it more difficult to get into the car, they locked all four doors, essentially negating the possibility that the piece of paper may fall out. They didn't consider that and began to make their way down Meeting Street.

They were looking for a relatively cheap clothing store for him and hers. After at least ten blocks they found no such store. Returning via the opposite one-way street, they did discover a store that had clothing for men and women. The clothing was not terribly overpriced and they each bought a new outfit. They went back to their room and made love, slowly.

"Honey," Jackie whispered into Robin's ear, "let's talk a little bit about our future. What are the things we can control and those we cannot?"

"You know," she whispered back to him, "I've just been thinking about where we go from here, but, first things first, we have to take you to a doctor to find out why you are having these frequent headaches. Have they gotten worse?"

"The answer to that is, yes, they have gotten progressively worse and recently have begun to throb continuously."

"OK, let's check with the landlady and find out the nearest doctor's office that she has some familiarity with," Robin stated with conviction.

"Ms. Robinson," Jackie queried, "we need to see a doctor who specializes in neurological diseases. Can you help us?"

"Dr. Moreland, I can tell you where there is a multispecialty clinic, but I'm not sure about doctors who specialize in neurological diseases," Ms. Robinson answered.

"That's fine," Jackie said, "tell us how to get to the clinic—is it nearby?"

"Well, I don't know. Are you walking?"

"Yes, we would like to walk," Robin said, adding to the conversation.

"OK, the clinic is near the medical school and hospital—about three blocks over and, I would say, nearly ten blocks up," Ms. Robinson said.

"Ms. Robinson," Robin said, "thank you for your recommendation and directions."

"You are most welcome and I'll look after your room—you don't mind if I do a little straightening up in there."

"Absolutely not," Jackie spoke up and added, "That would be great."

They walked three blocks over and actually twelve blocks up before they found the clinic. It was a large building with an equally large reception and waiting area. They paused to look at the physician directory.

"Hello, what can I do for you?" the receptionist asked, noticing they were looking at the directory.

Jackie spoke up first, "Yes, Ma'me, I need to see a doctor who specializes in neurological diseases."

"No problem, we have several neurologists—what is your specific problem?"

"Headaches."

"OK, let me recommend Dr. Sterling, a neurologist who sees all cases of persistent headaches—would you say it is persistent?"

"Yes, I would," Jackie answered, "and it has gotten progressively worse over the course of several days."

"Dr. Sterling has an opening at eleven o'clock this morning," the receptionist said and added, "You will have to see a triage nurse, in case you need x-rays or lab studies. Please have a seat and I will notify the nurse—it shouldn't be but a few minutes. In the meantime, you need to fill out this questionnaire about your symptoms, the medicines you take, and your past medical history."

"Thank you," they said simultaneously.

"Yes, Ma'me," Jackie answered.

"The triage nurse will see you now. Go into the first room on the left."

"Mr. and Mrs. Ferrell, I'm the triage nurse, Mrs. Singletary. Mr. Ferrell, before I take your vital signs, please describe your headaches for me."

"Well, I have suffered some rather severe headaches over the last four or five days."

"OK, I understand that, but give me a detailed description of the headaches."

"They are rather slow in coming on, but when they do, they are persistent and lately have been throbbing," Jackie replied.

"Have you taken anything for them and, if so, what?" she asked.

"Yes, Tylenol."

"How much Tylenol?"

"Two tablets every four hours or so—I think they are five hundred milligrams a piece," Jackie answered.

"Does that ease the pain?"

"No, it never knocks the headaches out completely," Jackie replied.

"Has anybody in your family complained of headaches?"

"Yes, my mother has."

"It says here she saw a doctor for a brain tumor," she noted.

"Yes, she had an astrocytoma removed surgically from the right side of her brain. It was superficial and rested over the right hemisphere, and the surgeon was able to excise the whole tumor with a rim of uninvolved tissue. This was followed by irradiation, but she did not receive chemotherapy. She has done well and was practically free of symptoms after several months of rehabilitation," Jackie explained.

The nurse asked, "Are your headaches localized?"

He answered with a question, "What do you mean by 'localized'?"

"Do they occur in a specific location, like over the left eye?"

"My headaches are diffuse, but they do seem to be worse over the left side," Jackie answered.

"One other thing: have you had any other symptoms like muscular weakness or difficulty seeing or hearing?"

"No, I have not."

The triage nurse hesitated, seeming to be thinking about something, and then she declared, "With this history and you specific set of symptoms, we will need to get some x-rays before you see the doctor. Are you allergic to x-ray dyes?"

"No, not that I know of," Jackie said. He was becoming aware of the fact that the nurse was concerned he might have something in his head like his mother had.

"Have you ever had an MRI?" she asked.

"No, not that I know of, but I really don't know what that is," he answered.

"It stands for 'Magnetic Resonance Imaging,'" she explained and added, "It's a sophisticated x-ray contrast study that clearly defines changes in the brain such as the presence of a brain tumor."

The nurse took Jackie's pulse, respirations, blood pressure, and temperature. She noted, "Your vital signs are all normal. Now let me take you down to x-ray for an x-ray of your lungs and a MRI of your brain."

After the x-rays were performed, Jackie and Robin were placed in a standard examination room to wait for the headache specialist, Dr.

Sterling. He came into the room, introduced himself, took a detailed medical history, and made an extensive physical examination.

"Mr. Ferrell," the doctor announced, "I have seen your x-rays and I am sorry to tell you that you have a brain tumor."

Jackie was dumbfounded, but able to ask, "Is it like the tumor my mother had?"

"It could be, but we won't know for sure what it is until we get a piece of the tumor and submit it to pathology for a definitive diagnosis," Dr. Sterling answered and added, "but also, I'm afraid there is a problem with the size and location of the tumor—"

Jackie didn't let him finish the sentence and blurted out, "What? How so?"

"Well, first of all, the tumor is large, about the size of a baseball, and, second of all, it is deep in the middle of the brain. I'm not a neurosurgeon, but my best guess is that it is inoperable—we wouldn't be able to get it all, if we operate. And then a neurosurgeon probably won't know for sure until the tumor is exposed—that is, if he can expose it. I might add, I'm surprised you haven't had more symptoms related to the central and deep location."

Jackie almost screamed, "Oh, my God, doctor, I'm only thirty-three years old...how can I have an inoperable brain tumor?"

Robin teared up when Jackie remonstrated.

"I know it may seem to be unusual to have a brain tumor at your age, but they do occur and, unfortunately, they are sometimes aggressive," Dr. Sterling said, emphasizing the word "aggressive."

"What will happen next?" Jackie said, barely able to see out of teary eyes.

"Well, first of all, you have to see a neurosurgeon who will decide whether or not the tumor is operable," he answered and added, "I am going to refer you to Dr. Castlewhite, a very well-respected neurosurgeon."

Dr. Castlewhite, a relatively young man in a long-length, starched, white "doctor" coat buttoned to the top where there was a bright red tie and white shirt, examined Jackie, made a review of symptoms and took a lengthy medical history. They reviewed the MRI together and Dr. Castlewhite made a distressing pronouncement.

"Your tumor is inoperable, but it may be sensitive to irradiation, so we will start there: irradiation every other day for two weeks and then a repeat MRI, approximately one month after the irradiation, assuming you have no intervening crisis such as brain swelling and/or enlargement of the tumor with additional symptoms. It is important for you to keep a positive attitude, get plenty of rest, and maintain a healthy intake of food and fluids. My secretary will make an appointment in radiology for you as soon as possible."

"Doctor, you didn't tell me the prognosis for this type of tumor," Jackie spoke in a quivering voice.

"I would think," Dr. Castlewhite said, "in six months, you will need hospice care, and it is unlikely you will live more than fifteen months." He, then, added, "You'll need to notify all your family members and put all your personal affairs in order."

Jackie lowered his head, shuttered, and tried to hold back the oncoming tears. Robin cried openly.

"Oh, God, Robin we'll have to call home and tell Caroline, Bill, and our folks," Jackie blurted out, surprised he could get any words out.

It was dark outside when Jackie dialed the Statesville number for Caroline, who answered after second ring.

"Caroline Moreland."

"Caroline, Jackie."

"Jackie, where have you been? Someone said you were in Charleston," Caroline asked.

"Yes, Robin and I are at a clinic near the Medical College of South Carolina here in Charleston. I'm afraid I have some bad news: I have been diagnosed with an inoperable brain tumor and have been told I have no more than fifteen months to live. I have scheduled to have irradiation of my brain right away. I'd like you to tell the children. After they release me when the irradiation is finished, and I have no acute problems, I'm going to come home and prepare myself for hospice care. I'll stay with my parents until then. That should give you time to prepare the children and to decide whether or not you and the children want to see me," Jackie said, almost out of breath.

"Oh, God, Jackie, I'm so sorry to hear your sad news," Caroline responded and added, "I will tell the children when I think the time is right, because I know they'll want to see you either before or after hospice care."

"Thank you, Caroline, have the children call me at my folks if they want to talk to me and maybe I can help them understand what's brought me back home," Jackie concluded the call.

He then turned the phone over to Robin, who phoned home.

Bill answered, "Bill Smithwick."

"Bill, Robin," she said, trying to keep her voice from faltering.

"Robin, my gosh, it seems like months since I talked to you—how are you?"

"I'm fine, Bill, but Jackie has been diagnosed with an inoperable brain tumor," she said, pausing to collect herself." She continued, "He will have to have irradiation and if he is stable after that, we are coming home for hospice care."

"Oh, God, I'm sorry to hear that," Bill replied in a genuine tone of voice.

"Thank you," she responded, and added, "I'll leave it up to you what you tell the children, if anything, and decide whether or not you and/or the children want to see me. Jackie will stay with his folks until he's admitted to hospice."

'I appreciate the heads-up on this, and please call me again when you get back home," Bill replied, realizing—at long last—there were more important things than your wife having an affair.

Both Robin and Jackie realized, being hopeful, that the lawsuits were now null and void. Also the divorce decrees would have surely been put on the back burner, but that had not been confirmed. Robin then called her aunt and uncle.

"William Smithwick, here," her uncle answered.

"Uncle William, this is Robin, I need to tell you something very important," she said.

Her uncle paused briefly, sighed, and said, "Go ahead, shoot."

"Jackie has been having headaches that really didn't respond to analgesics. We decided to go have it checked out, and we went to a neurologist and who examined him and took an MRI x-ray of his head. He discovered a brain tumor and referred us to a neurosurgeon to see if it could be removed. The surgeon told us, unfortunately, that the tumor could not be removed and recommended two weeks of irradiation. After that he will come home and be admitted at some point in time to hospice care here in Statesville," she stopped, took a deep breath, and waited for her uncle's response.

"Robin, I'm very sorry to hear that, and while you are still in Charleston, why don't you stay with us? You have rented a car, haven't you?" her uncle asked.

"Oh, Uncle William, that would be wonderful. Thank you for your support," she said with a lilt in her voice, and then added, "We'll be there tomorrow after his first round of irradiation."

It became unusually cool as the night descended. It was one of those nights when the moon and stars shone brightly, indicating a clear sky for a clear night. Jackie and Robin drove back to the bed and breakfast—glad they had some new clothes. They had stopped at a McDonald's for a quick snack, so food was not on their minds and neither was sex. They undressed quickly and silently and went straight to bed—cuddling for a while before sleep overtook them.

The next morning, they were hungry and they had a big breakfast. After checking out of the bed and breakfast, they headed back to the clinic for Jackie's first set of x-ray therapies. Then they made their way back to Robin's aunt and uncle's place to relax and rest. They paused for a while to make conversation with Aunt Stacy.

"Many thanks for allowing us to stay with you again," Robin said and added, "we're afraid we will not be much company these next few days."

"We're so sorry," her aunt responded. "This has got to be a big shock to you both."

Robin paused to get her breath and replied, "Absolutely, what has happened to us puts a new twist on our life; it capsules time down to a few months. This makes you realize what is really important in life and makes you begin to think about the hereafter. How much will Jackie suffer, I have no idea, but we have to be prepared for the worst and hope for the best. And to top it all off, we have to have some sort of reconciliation with our families in Statesville. We have already alerted them to what has happened, when we will be coming back and where we will stay."

"Well, you can certainly stay here as long as you like or as long as you need to," her aunt replied.

"Again, thank you. I'm certain you will have your reward for taking us in and providing us a place to rest, relax, and put our life in some kind of order," Robin said, feeling genuinely grateful.

They excused themselves and went to their room. Jackie was surprised as to how much the irradiation had taken out of him. He was exhausted. He napped and Robin read a romance novel her aunt had left in the room. It was very quiet in the house and warm in the bedroom. She was thankful for being near family when the crisis hit. Robin was also thankful for the quiet and comfort of the room. Between chapters she watched Jackie sleep; she was warmed by the touch of his body. For her, life had begun anew and felt different somehow—she sensed the calmness in her body and soul that was not there before. As calming as the surroundings were, she still steeled herself for whatever came next and for the expected rapid loss of life of the man by her side. The fear of being caught and having to go home and face the music was quelled by the present circumstances. She hardly considered the fact that there might be people out there looking for them. Something like that was hardly significant when you were facing death.

The weather turned bad for the fall quarter. There was intermittent rain that settled in for days—the sun ducked behind the clouds and remained there. Darkness began to come down earlier after the fall equinox. As if the times were not depressive enough, the weather just added to the misery and heartache of Jackie and Robin. The weeks of irradiation limped by and Jackie got progressively weaker, and, with no appetite, was unable to keep his weight and energy up—on top of that his mental depression remained inexorable. Robin could not keep him from getting down emotionally, but she somehow kept his head above water, helping him maintain a positive attitude. Her aunt and uncle were consistently supportive—they had read up on brain tumors and the treatment of patients near the end of life. They were made aware of the possible complications in a large, inoperable brain tumor. As a result of the irradiation, they learned the tumor could actually en-large rather than shrink due to necrosis and/or bleeding. As time went by, it was apparent that the tumor would likely put pressure on the ventricular system and cause increased intracerebral pressure, which would necessitate placing a catheter in one of the ventricles. Finally, it was apparent that infection would become a real possibility.

To the surprise of all, Jackie and Robin got handwritten notes from Caroline and Bill, expressing their heartfelt love and concern for Jackie—it was a life-changing response from their heart-broken former mates. They knew, then, they could go home and be received unconditionally, but not necessarily with open arms. After all that had happened, it was, to them, nothing short of a miracle—Jackie's de-pression eased off, and both of them knew they could approach his death with calm and dignity.

One night after they had received the incredibly supportive notes, Robin, in the face of the usual quiet after irradiation, said, "Honey, you know what?"

"What?"

"I'm going to respond to the notes both of them have written."

"You know I thought about that, but I didn't think it would be the wisest thing to do, since we have long been in a small doghouse, having caused a hurt that would have been irrevocable," Jackie said in a quiet husky voice.

"Well, my thought was that no matter how badly they were hurt, they had responded to our phone calls, leaving the hurt and bitterness on the shelf, and it would be an equally unexpected response on our part, if we wrote both of them notes," Robin expounded.

"You know, Robin, it certainly couldn't hurt and it might be received with the same spirit they exhibited when they sent their notes," Jackie surmised, turning his thoughts around in a positive fashion.

They didn't say it, but they both hoped their action might just pave the way for reconciliation between them and their former spouses.

Except for extreme weakness and loss of appetite, Jackie finished the irradiation to his brain without any other serious side effects. The tumor was said to have been reduced in size by nearly fifty percent. The doctors were confident there would not be any swelling of the brain with increased intracranial I pressure.

He and Robin, anxious and a bit scared, prepared themselves for the long trip home to Statesville. Robin drove and during the trip, as the landscape went by, they talked a great deal about what to expect going home.

She noted with genuine affect, "Honey, I don't know about you, but I am relieved to be going home. There's no way we can predict the reception we will receive, but I think we have laid the ground work for at least some degree of reconciliation—I imagine there will be different degrees of sympathy, or should I say empathy."

"I'm with you, babe, but I just hope, before I die, I can gain some of my energy back and enjoy the last days of my life," Jackie, in the front passenger's seat in a reclining setting, responded to Robin's thoughts.

She let that comment sink in a little and said, "Oh, God, I too hope you can enjoy your last days. I do know in hospice there is almost always pain control and I bet your head is going to hurt, but to what degree nobody seems to know. It is always related to how each individual handles the pain that almost always accompanies cancer."

"Well," he came back rather quickly, "the one thing I am concerned about is whether or not we will be allowed to stay together."

"I know what you mean, but don't you think I'll be able to stay with you in hospice?" she asked.

"No doubt you'll be able to stay with me during the daylight hours, but I don't think it would be prudent to stay overnight—certainly it might be poorly received and, frankly the staff probably wouldn't allow it," he answered and added, "Robin, you and I need to talk to my parents and plan a funeral or a memorial service."

"Gosh, Jackie, I really haven't thought much about that, but you're right, it has to be done, the sooner the better," she responded, fighting back fresh tears.

At that silence prevailed and monotony set in. Actually, Robin was relieved to be busy driving, combating the silence and monotony. She took Interstate ninety-five past Fayetteville and then took a ramp onto Interstate forty, the highway that would take them to Statesville.

It was October and the leaves were turning and beginning to fall. The weatherman was correct when he said that the heat of summer was over, but he didn't anticipate Indian summer, which could bring in some very warm days. Unconcerned about the weather, Jackie and Robin went straight to the hospice unit and checked in.

The receptionist received them warmly with "Welcome to hospice. Are you here to visit or are you going to be a patient?"

"I'm going to be a patient, but I don't think I am quite ready. Did you get referral papers from the clinic in Charleston?" Jackie answered.

"What is your name?" she asked, leafing through a stack of papers.

"Jackie Moreland, or it could be Jack Ferrell," he responded.

"Yes, we have referral papers on you. I can see you are not ready for hospice just yet," she noted, but added, "We still would like for you to check in with our nurse on duty and get baseline vital signs and a history of symptoms."

"I agree—I think that would be a good idea; then I can be ready to be admitted to hospice when the time comes," Jackie said.

The receptionist punched a button on her phone and said, "Mrs. Stafford, I have a patient here who has been referred here from a clinic in Charleston, South Carolina. We have received referral papers and I have told the patient, Dr. Jackie Moreland, he should present himself to you for baseline vital signs and a symptoms review."

"Of course, send him in," the nurse responded.

"Dr. Moreland, go to the second door on the right. Mrs. Stafford is waiting for you."

Jackie went to the second door on the right and introduced himself and Robin to Mrs. Stafford.

"Dr. Moreland, let me see your papers before I take your vitals and review your symptoms," Mrs. Stafford said in a very professional manner. She looked through the papers and said, "These papers are in order. Please step on the scales and we'll get your weight. That's one hundred sixty pounds. How much many pounds have you lost?" she asked.

"Between ten and fifteen," Jackie said.

"OK, we'll monitor that for the rest of the time you're here. As you know, your weight is an important indicator of how your condition is progressing, or should I say digressing."

"I understand that, but you know I have very little appetite," Jackie pointed out.

"Oh, yes, Dr. Moreland, that's to be expected in your situation. Now let me get your vital signs."

Mrs. Stafford moved on and took his blood pressure, respirations, pulse, and temperature. She noted his vital signs were within normal range, except for his body temperature, which was a degree above normal.

"Dr. Moreland, you temperature is slightly above normal. I'm going to ask you to take your temperature daily before you eat or drink anything. Keep a record of that and bring it with you the next time you come.

"Now, what are you to expect? First of all, your appetite will probably not get any better. Secondly, as the tumor progresses you will probably get more headaches related to increased intracranial pressure. The headaches could be associated with nausea and vomiting. Thirdly, some patients with your diagnosis get a syndrome with diarrhea. You have to be very careful you do not get dehydrated. We can treat most of you symptoms, but eventually you will have to go on morphine to sedate you and keep you comfortable and free of pain. At some point it is likely you will lose consciousness."

"Mrs. Stafford, what is the drill? When will I know it's time to come in?"

"You can stay home as long as you are comfortable and free of unremitting pain," Mrs. Stafford responded, and then added, "Incidentally, someone from this unit will check on you daily, so don't worry, we'll know when it's time for you to come in."

"I'm going to stay with my parents, Dr. and Mrs. Moreland, who have a home on Dogwood Circle," Jackie said.

"OK, good, just leave your address and phone number with our receptionist and we will follow you closely," Mrs. Stafford explained.

"I'll do that, and I appreciate you telling me how my symptoms will progress as I live out my last days," Jackie responded.

Jackie called home and his mother answered, "The Moreland residence."

"Mom, this is Jackie."

"Jackie, dear, where are you?" she asked.

Jackie answered, "Robin and I are in Statesville."

"Robin? Who is Robin?" she asked, seemingly unaware of the relationship that had been going on for some time.

"Mom, don't you know? Surely you and Dad have heard about my affair with Robin Smithwick," Jackie said, incredulous and dumbfounded.

"Oh, yes, I heard about it, but I have chosen to ignore it like it never happened," his mom said casually.

"Well," Jackie pressed on, "it has happened—it is very real and you have to face it," Jackie replied, a forceful, but respectful, tone to his voice.

"I've heard you have some kind of brain tumor," she said, abruptly changing the subject.

"Yes, the tumor is inoperable and I have just finished irradiation treatments. I am now under hospice care, but until things get worse, I'd like to stay with you and Dad."

"And Robin, is she going to stay here?"

"Yes, she is going to stay with me, if you and Dad don't mind—she is an important part of my life and I'm not going to let us be separated. Is that OK?" he asked, suddenly feeling like he was going to be rejected.

"I don't know, son, I'll have to discuss it with your father," she said dismissively and added a question, "Aren't you still married to Caroline?"

"Mother, Caroline and I are separated and she has filed for a divorce. So we are married in name only," Jackie replied, rapidly running out of patience. He didn't wait for any response and added, "I will call you tomorrow to find out what your decision is." He hung up.

Next, Robin called Bill, who, surprisingly, was at home.

"Bill, Robin."

"Oh, hello, Robin, I heard you were back in town."

She gasped, absolutely amazed at how fast news traveled, especially bad news, and said, "I guess you remember about Jackie having an inoperable brain tumor."

"Yes, I do, and I am sorry to hear that. What's going to happen?" he asked, not very sensitive to the situation.

"Well, Jackie has already signed up for hospice and will be monitored on a daily basis. In the meantime, we are hoping to stay with his folks until he is admitted to the hospice unit for his last days," Robin tearfully explained.

"What about you?" he asked, not quite over the fact Robin had had an affair with one of his best friends.

"I'm going to be by his side until the very end," Robin said, with emphasis on the word "end," and added, "I would like to see the kids, if that is possible."

"I'll discuss this with the children...they already know about Jackie being sick," Bill responded.

The next step was to call Caroline, who answered on the first ring, "Moreland residence."

"Caroline, this is Jackie."

"Jackie, I know about your illness...how are you doing?"

"As good as could be expected, I guess," Jackie said, a little dejection in his voice.

"Are you back in town?" she asked.

"Yes, we're back and I'm hoping to stay with my folks until it's time to go into the hospice unit. Before I get any worse, I'd like to see the kids," Jackie said, a hopeful edge to his voice.

"Jackie, we have adjusted to life without you and I'm not sure about you seeing the children," Caroline reacted with some finality.

"Well, I understand that. How about I call you tomorrow...I would hope you would discuss this with the kids. As an aside, I want to thank you for your note—it meant a lot."

"You are certainly welcome and I will talk to you tomorrow," Caroline said and closed the line.

Jackie had two people to talk to and he wasn't very excited about it, because he was afraid of the possible reaction to the presence of Robin in his life. He started with Caroline.

She answered the phone with two rings. "The Morelands."

"Caroline, Jackie."

"Jackie, I am so sorry to say that the kids and I are well beyond any association with you, so you won't be able to see the kids," Caroline said with conviction and added quickly, "Goodbye and good luck."

"Caroline, does that mean you and the children will not attend my memorial service?"

Robin didn't wait for Bill to call. She dialed his phone the day after their conversation about the children. It was after work, so she could be sure to get bill at home.

"The Smithwick residence," Bill answered.

"Bill, Robin."

"Robin, I haven't had any time to talk to the kids, but I know what the answer will be: the kids and I have moved on without you in our life—we aren't interested in starting all over with you suddenly in our lives again."

"OK, thanks, Bill," Robin responded sadly, but, then added, "does that mean you and the children will not attend my memorial service?"

"Well, honey, I can tell by the way the conversation went you will not be allowed to see the kids," Jackie observed with equal sadness.

"Baby, we are rebuffed at every turn—I am honestly not surprised, but I wonder if this is not a message for us to pack up and head out of town," Robin surmised.

"Robin, we cannot leave town without having hospice available," Jackie came to Robin.

"I understand that, but hospice would be available almost anywhere we would happen to go, particularly if the town we settle in is large enough to have that service," Robin said with some intensity.

"I have an idea—and you will think I'm crazy—what about going to a state that has liberal end-of-life laws?" Jackie responded with a little lilt in his voice.

"Wait a minute, what are you trying to say?" Robin responded, suddenly reacting to Jackie's implication they go to a state in which there is a law legalizing physician-assisted suicide.

"You're a sharp girl, you know exactly what I'm saying," Jackie responded.

"Are you suggesting we go to Oregon?"

"No, to Vermont, where they just passed a physician-assisted suicide initiative. It would be the closest and it wouldn't cost us an arm and a leg to get there," Jackie answered with positive conviction.

"If you go, I'm going!" Robin said, her voice rising, but cracking.

"Well, there is no doubt about that," Jackie responded.

"And, if you sign up for assisted suicide, why can't I join you?"

"Robin," Jackie said with exasperation in his voice, "you can't talk like that—you can't mean it—I'm the one who's dying!"

"Jackie, you are my life—if you are going to kill yourself, I am, too."

"Oh, Lord, Robin," Jackie lamented, "What am I going to do with you?"

"Love me as you always have," Robin closed the conversation.

Jackie looked in the encyclopedia for the largest town in Vermont and selected Burlington as their destination. He then called Mrs. Stafford at the Statesville hospice unit.

"Statesville Hospice," the receptionist answered.

"Mrs. Stafford, please," Jackie requested.

"Please hold the line while I get Mrs. Stafford for you."

"This is Mrs. Stafford."

"Mrs. Stafford, this is Jackie Moreland...I need to tell you about a decision Robin and I have made."

"OK, I have a feeling this is going to be monumental, go ahead."

"We have decided to go to Burlington, Vermont, apply for end-of-life care, and consider assisted suicide."

"Oh, my, this is monumental—and you need me to get the papers together and pave the way for you to go to Vermont."

"Exactly," Jackie said.

"OK, I appreciate your decision and I will not judge it at all and I will talk to the hospice unit in Burlington—you come over here early in the morning and I will have everything ready for you." Mrs. Stafford replied.

"Thank you, Mrs. Stafford," Jackie said and added, "we are most appreciative for all you have done for us. If you tell me your address, I will send you a note concerning our decision to avoid undue suffering and ask for help in dying."

Things were moving rapidly—the holidays were upon them and Jackie and Robin were on the road again. They had a contact person in Vermont at Burlington Hospice, a Mrs. Johnson. They once again had a rent-a-car, a Chevrolet Malibu that had more pep than any car they had had before. Despite the rain, they made good time going up Interstate ninety-five. They had planned on at least one stop in

Delaware, before they pushed on to Vermont. They were to go straight to hospice and check in with Mrs. Johnson—the hospice unit was not hard to find.

Jackie had easily convinced Robin to not mention suicide, even though his symptoms, which had been outline by Mrs. Stafford, had steadily increased, particularly his headaches, anorexia, nausea, and fatigue. His mood swings had stopped—he was persistently depressed. In his depressed state, of course, suicide was looking more and more like a reality. And to top it off, it was snowing in Vermont and, of course, that was both a blessing and a curse—there was no need to drive, so they turned the car in before the roads became impassable, impassable for a southerner.

Robin and Jackie trekked through the snow to the Hospice Center of Burlington, the largest city in Vermont. They were received warmly by a receptionist.

"Good afternoon, welcome to the Hospice Center of Burlington."

"We are here to see Mrs. Johnson, who, I hope, has received referral papers from the hospice unit in Statesville, North Carolina," Jackie announced in a rather deep, raspy voice—he looked emaciated.

"Please have a seat and get Mrs. Johnson for you," the receptionist responded.

Both of them had donned winter clothes and they were relieved to be able to shed their jackets.

Jackie, after the trek, was winded, weak, and suffering a severe headache. He was thirsty, but not hungry.

Mrs. Johnson, with papers, appeared in front of them and said, "Dr. Moreland and Mrs. Smithwick, welcome to our hospice unit."

Jackie responded, "Thank you, we are glad to be here, even if we are not used to such snow."

"Now, Dr. Moreland, I have reviewed your papers from Statesville and I am aware of you situation, but I do need to get some baseline vital signs and a review of your symptoms before we go any further," Mrs. Johnson, a grey-haired women in a nurse's uniform, stated. She added, "Come with me and we'll go into one of the examination rooms."

She checked Jackie's pulse, blood pressure, respirations, and temperature and stated, "Your pulse is slightly up, your blood pressure is down a bit, your respirations are just above normal, and your temperature is increased by a degree and a half. Now, how far did you and Mrs. Smithwick walk in the snow?"

"I don't know, but I'm guessing it was several miles," Jackie responded.

"Well," Mrs. Johnson said, "some of these changes in your vital signs may be related to that trek you just made. What I would like to do is repeat these vitals once everything has settled down. Now, after all that, please tell me how you were doing before your outdid yourself in the snow."

"Well, Mrs. Johnson, as you can surely tell, I am not doing very well—I have no appetite, I stay nauseated, I am getting progressively weaker, my headaches are severe, and, as you can imagine, I don't sleep well at all," Jackie summarized his symptoms.

"Do you have any other symptoms? I presume you stay depressed," Mrs. Johnson asked.

"I'm having some loose stools, spots are forming before my eyes, and, as you note, I am depressed," Jackie added.

"All right, I think these symptoms are serious and unremitting, and I recommend you be admitted to our hospice unit and sedated so that you can get some rest and not experience any more suffering."

"Mrs. Johnson, it is obvious that I am at the end of my days on this earth. I want to be in control of my own death. Realistically, then, are there choices available to me, so that I can determine the end of my life?"

"Dr. Moreland," Mrs. Johnson responded, "at this stage in your life and considering the degree of discomfort you are experiencing, I would say there are three choices and they are somewhat related due to the fact that we have to keep you free of unremitting pain: 1) you chose to be sedated to just before you would experience unconsciousness; 2) you chose to be sedated to unconsciousness as food and water are removed from your treatment regimen; 3) you chose physician-assisted suicide and have complete control of your death."

"So, you're telling me I am a candidate for physician-assisted suicide?"

"You very well may be, but you have to be seen and evaluated by two of our doctors—I think they would want to address your degree of depression and determine if you are in a rational state of mind. Do you know exactly what you are doing by asking to be put to sleep permanently?" she asked.

"Mrs. Johnson, yes, I do—to tell you the truth, in all aspects, I am more than ready. In consideration of the choices you laid out for me, I think physician-assisted suicide best fits my view of how I want to die. For me this decision is also complicated by Mrs. Smithwick's desire to die in the same mode as I. That is to say we want to die simultaneously, and the only way to do that without any other complicating factors is to for us both to submit to physician-assisted suicide."

"Dr. Moreland, there is a huge problem with that decision: there is no precedent for such a maneuver and, therefore, a dual death by such a mode has no legal basis and I'm sure the physicians who pass on PAS would decline to participate in such an unusual death. They have no legal basis to back up such an unusual and unprecedented request, but just to cover all the bases I will pass the request onto the physicians in charge of the assisted suicide."

Two physicians, one of them a psychiatrist, examined Jackie and completed an exhausting review of symptoms. They determined that he was rational and completely aware of the seriousness of what he had decided to do. They were not surprised that he was depressed and weighed that in their decision. One of the physicians wrote an order for Jackie to receive chocolate pudding lased with a lethal dose of a short-acting barbiturate sedative. Neither of them was made aware of Robin's desire to be put to sleep also. The nurses felt the timing was not right to broach the subject.

It was not lost on either Jackie or Robin that they were considering something, not only illegal, but, in the history of Vermont medicine, also unprecedented. As Jackie frequently said, "It's a conundrum—maybe more than a simple conundrum."

Jackie asked Mrs. Johnson, "How long is the chocolate pudding good for?"

"I don't know, Dr. Moreland, we have never had to consider keeping the pudding beyond the day it was to be given."

"OK," he said, "tell the pharmacy to hold up the concoction until we can sort out this problem."

"Will do, but we will have to repeat the order whenever you are ready," Mrs. Johnson responded.

"Do you know any physician who would consider Mrs. Smithwick's request?" Jackie asked.

"I don't know," Mrs. Johnson opined and added, "I have not had any request like this—it might take me some time to do that."

"Mrs. Johnson, " Jackie persisted, "I don't want to tell you what to do, but maybe one of the examining physicians would be willing to order a second cocktail for Mrs. Smithwick."

"That might have some validity, if it is determined that Mrs. Swithwick is of sound mind, but, because of the circumstances, is in a state of depression. Her emotional attachment to you is obviously extremely strong, and apparently she sees no reason to live on in face of your death. I will contact the psychiatrist member of the examining physicians," Mrs. Johnson answered, willing to be as helpful as possible.

She knew she was dealing with a well-educated couple who have been hit with a devastating situation and that they were sincere in their desire to die together. It was a first, but Mrs. Johnson doubted it would be the last. She called the psychiatrist, a Dr. Jackson, and asked him if he would be available to examine Mrs. Smithwick with the thought of giving her a lethal cocktail.

Dr. Jackson replied immediately, "Absolutely not—it is not only illegal, but unprecedented."

Not to be deterred, Mrs. Johnson called the other member of the examining team, a Dr. Satterwhite, and asked, "Dr. Satterwhite, would you consider examining Mr. Moreland's paramour in consideration of giving her a cocktail at the same time as Moreland?"

"Not on your life, Mrs. Johnson. I'm not in the business of killing off perfectly healthy young people."

Mrs. Johnson appeared in Jackie's room and announced she had tried to get both doctors to prescribe a lethal cocktail for Mrs. Smithwick, but to no avail—they didn't even take the time to think about it.

"Honey, it looks like we are back to square one—no place to turn to, no way to get out of a compelling situation," Jackie said to Robin.

Robin shuttered and broke into convulsive crying. Even in such a state, even after all that had happened, Robin was still one of the most beautiful women he had ever seen.

He added, "Well, I'm not giving up."

Robin broke into his reverie, "Honey, you've read up on some of this—aren't there other ways to lose consciousness and pass onto the other side?"

Jackie was quiet for a few moments and asked, "Do you have something specific in mind?"

"Yes, instead of a double suicide, we could stage a homicide just before the suicide."

"Are you crazy? Are you suggesting that I commit murder before I commit suicide?" Jackie asked, incredulously.

"Yes, as they say, I am deadly serious," Robin spoke in a very firm, positive tone of voice.

"Well, do tell me how I am supposed to kill you off," Jackie said sarcastically. He thought that there was no way, even if Robin was mentally and emotionally prepared to be killed, he could do it.

Robin knew how it could be done and done humanely, i.e., cover her face with a pillow, but she knew she needed to do some more persuading. She tried again to convince Jackie that this was the way to go, but to no avail.

Late fall in Vermont was spectacular, a veritable maze of color—golds, reds, yellows, and browns—and when they fell the leaves produced a classic mixture of the incredible colors produced by nature's mysteries—that is, when the ground wasn't covered by a foot or so of snow.

Robin stayed and slept in Jackie's room and when awake, she listened to his murmuring at a soft level consistent with his state of sedation. He was, if not happy, in a comfortable state of semiconsciousness, yet able to respond to the constant touches from Robin. Jackie was able to administer the morphine at his own pace, able to determine his own need, which was to avoid pain at all costs.

A nurse stepped into the room at regular intervals, checking on the status of her patient. Finally, at Jackie's request, Mrs. Johnson came in with the lethal cocktail, giving him the chocolate pudding in a cup with a spoon. To no one in particular, Jackie commented that it appeared to be a large amount of pudding, but he began to eat the pudding as directed.

The nurse stayed in to monitor the patient's reaction to the cocktail and to determine the patient's time of death. He rapidly lost consciousness and the ability to eat the pudding, leaving the remaining part of the mixture untouched. Mrs. Johnson took his pulse and listened to his heart and, when the beating stopped, pronounced him dead at 2:20 in the afternoon. Inexplicably, she did not recover the cup and spoon.

Now, the room was dark and Robin had been allowed to lie on the bed with Jackie and she recovered the cocktail and proceeded to finish the pudding, the cup and spoon falling between the two lovers. No more than ten minutes after Jackie died, Robin did also. Mrs. Johnson was shocked to find the empty cup on Robin's side of the bed—she realized her mistake and was mortified. She knew then she had to notify the medical examiner, who would have to submit a report on the death of both persons. The one report of a physician-assisted suicide was straight-forward, the laws of Vermont had accounted for such a suicide and it was reported as such.

At first it seemed the death of Robin Smithwick was a different matter, but because it was intentional, it was also ruled a suicide. The medical examiner was not privy to the fact that the cup was empty and left in the bed between the two bodies. Mrs. Johnson was devastated, but, as time went by, it became apparent to her colleagues that, yes, she appeared to be careless, but down deep she, too, was intentional. Further, as more time went by, it became known to all who cared that the pharmacist was also intentional. No criminal charges were brought forth onto the principal characters.

After embalming, the two bodies were shipped to Statesville, North Carolina, for a dual memorial service and burial in three days, allowing time for those family members who were coming from out of state to attend the service. Despite the circumstances, the service was well-attended and the audience included four children, who, despite a long preparatory discussion, were in a state of confusion and shock.

The Reverend Beverly Jackson from the First Presbyterian Church gave the homily declaring that only God could judge these two young people in their decision to commit suicide. He also stated that nowhere in the Bible did it declare that suicide was a sin. It was clear to the Reverend that Jackie and Robin had decided to live on the edge, thwarting the usual societal restraints that most of us live by. He went on to say that does not necessarily make them bad persons, just different, marching to the beat of a rare drummer.

Finally, he questioned: did this couple go to heaven and be with the Lord? It was a question that many interested persons would ask and yet, we could not know the answer. If you did answer the question, you had made a judgment decision. Dr. Jackson announced they would be buried side by side, knowing that was what they would have wanted. Approximately one-half of the attendees came to the burial service. There was a very poignant moment in the service when the Moreland and Smithwick children added dirt to the tops of both coffins. At that moment, the collective tears flowed ever more freely. Somehow, as time went by, the children of both families began to understand what happened to one of their parents.

It would be a long time before those affected by the double suicide would be able to carry on without the stigma the event perpetrated on each of them. Over time the family members and close friends would come to see the deaths of Jackie Moreland and Robin Smithwick the way one would see the deaths of Romeo and Juliet. That view was understandable, but it was likely that Shakespearian experts would only begrudge the superficial similarity of the two events. Death was considered the great equalizer, but there was something about Robin's and Jackie's lives that even death could not bring them down to earth.